inShape
inLove
inSpired!

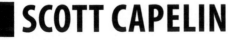 SCOTT CAPELIN

inShape

inLove

inSpired!

The 3 Step Wellness Blueprint for Using Peak
Health as The Foundation for Abundant Life

SCOTT CAPELIN

SCAN ME

inShape inLove inSpired!
The 3 Step Wellness Blueprint for Using Peak Health as The Foundation for Abundant Life
First Edition, 2021
ISBN: 979-8-4529012-0-4 (Amazon Print)
ISBN: 978-0-6452404-0-5 (IngramSpark Paperback)
ISBN: 978-0-6452404-1-2 (IngramSpark Hardcover)
ISBN: 978-1-0056978-9-1 (Smashwords)
ASIN: B099JZJZDF (e-Book)

Author Website: www.scottcapelin.co
Main Website: www.inlifecoaching.com.au
Publisher Website: www.evolveglobalpublishing.com

Table of Contents

About the Author 1

My Journey 5

About the Book.. 11

What Others Say About Scott 15

Introduction 19

Working With Scott... 27

Book Bonus.. 31

inShape...**33**

How To Approach Long-Term Health and Fitness 35

What Is Your WHY for Peak Health?.. 49

Accountability Makes Everything Happen Faster...................... 65

Weight Loss and Nutrition 75

What Type of Exercise Should I Do?..111

Fasting — The Ultimate Weight Loss and Health

Improvement Hack..121

How to Stay Motivated...127

The 80/20 Rule..137

inLove **141**

Your Relationship With Yourself 143

Identifying Your Values..157

Success Leaves Clues 175

Who Is Influencing You and How Are You Influencing

Yourself?..179

inSpired **189**

Passion and Purpose..191

The Courage to Change and Have a Go!.....................................205

Mindset Mastery...231

Curating Your Dream Life by Planning Perfect Days.................249

About the Author

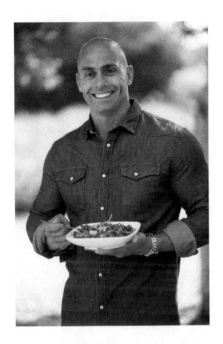

"I firmly believe that the universe directs us towards a place that we belong. I've had my fair share of ups and downs, and now I have a beautiful family and a thriving business and and I feel like I am exactly where I am supposed to be. If it was not for the hard times I've been through, I would not be where I am now, so I am grateful for them. I can see that everything really does happen for a reason"

~ Scott Capelin ~

A qualified wellness coach, nutritionist, and life coach with a Bachelor of Commerce, Scott Capelin comes to you having owned nine successful businesses over a 16-year period, with extensive business mentoring experience and over 20 years working with clients in the fitness industry and wellness arena.

By his own admission, however, Scott has also had his fair share of disappointment – losing one business, his livelihood and his family home while his wife was pregnant with their third child. Never one to give up, he worked to gain it all back, and more, within two years.

1

Seeing his role as helping others achieve a healthy, happy lifestyle through balancing family, fitness and finances, Scott Capelin is passionate about providing advice and encouragement as someone who has 'been there and done that!'

To my wife, Lauren. Thank you for your unwavering support and belief in me.

Thank you for your love, strength and courage.

I admire you more than you will ever know.

I love the way you believe that anything is possible.

Thank you for partnering with me through this life. It is truly an honour to be your man.

Thank you to the thousands of people who have given me permission to help them with their goal to live healthier and more fulfilling life.

Your journey has also been mine, and I have learned as much from you as you have from me.

▌ My Journey

After high school, I completed a business degree and entered the corporate world. I didn't mind the work, however, I couldn't see myself there for the next few decades.

My colleagues worked long hours, often in roles that I felt weren't meaningful, and I noticed their health and family lives suffered as they climbed the corporate ladder.

Whilst in that job, I studied to obtain my fitness industry qualifications. In my corporate role in 1998, when I asked my boss for time off and he said no, I knew I wouldn't be an employee for much longer.

I also worked pretty hard for two years and received a pay rise of only 4%, which took my annual salary from $37,000 to $38,480. It was time to make a move to doing something more fulfilling, and learn all the skills I need to be able to do it for myself.

Deep down I knew there must be a way to do work I love, with people I like, the way I want. I ditched the business suit to become a personal trainer.

I remember speaking to my dad about wanting to change. At that stage, I had completed a four-year Bachelor of Commerce degree at university and spent a further four years in the big business arena. Making a complete change to start from scratch and follow my passion, seemed like I would be wasting the best part of the previous decade.

I remember my dad taking a moment to pause as he thought. He said, "Just do whatever makes you happy". I am eternally grateful to him

5

for his support and advice, and the way that he and my mum were always there for me (and still are).

They never pushed me into anything. They supported me whenever I needed it. I made the career change and from day one, I absolutely loved it!

I moved into health club management and over the course of the next 20 years, ended up opening, building, and selling nine health clubs, two beauty salons, and a consulting business, not only in Australia but overseas as well.

I also studied to become a qualified nutritionist, Pilates instructor, NLP Practitioner, wellness advisor, and life purpose coach - all while coaching and mentoring many other individuals and business owners in the areas of health, business, and lifestyle coaching.

Your dream job does not exist.

You must create it.

What I have discovered throughout my time as a health and lifestyle coach, entrepreneur and business mentor is the lack of balance in people's lives, poor awareness regarding the things that make them truly happy, never-ending stress, limited time, an ongoing search for passion and meaning, and minimal awareness regarding the requirements to build truly powerful relationships around them.

I learned the hard way how little I knew about many of these areas too. I witnessed people with loads of money who were miserable or in poor health; people with great health who hated their work; and people struggling in relationships that couldn't seem to light the flame within.

I worked with people in a health and business coaching capacity who thought they wanted to lose weight or make more money, but on a deeper level, they just wanted to get more out of life. They wanted more happiness. On a broader level, they sought more fulfilment.

And, at the most basic level, they wanted more peace because their angst stemmed from living a life that wasn't in alignment with who they truly were or what they really wanted.

They say coaches and speakers often cover the topics they need most themselves. It's almost like the coach has a dark side and as a result, a coach sometimes feels like an impostor because they are not perfect. However, hopefully, the imperfections make them relatable; they certainly make a coach empathetic.

The aim is to shine a light on the darkness in the hope the coach can help other people who may be struggling with the same issues. I've had a lot of success and my fair share of failures, and I have definitely learned a lot more from the failures.

I've never had much trouble staying in shape. However, over the course of my life, I've had to do a lot of work addressing my relationships and the people I associate with, the way I look at life, my goals and life path, and ultimately, the decisions I make. I've been down the wrong road a few times and made poor decisions.

As a result, I've gained a great deal of clarity and wisdom regarding the life I want to live and the qualities I want to espouse. I want to help other people in these areas because I understand the power and conviction that can be attained by understanding exactly who you are, what you want and how to get it.

Through my own life journey, I've realised that my primary goal is to help people maximise opportunities to live a healthy life with passion, purpose, and positive relationships.

Nothing sums up my goal more than my experience with Matt. Matt was a 140-kilogram accountant who worked to lose 50 kilograms and ended up becoming a successful mentor in his own right. It was Matt's health and weight that initially acted as the catalyst for change in his life. Ultimately, this led to the confidence to change careers and go on to meet the woman he married.

Life balance, health, and relationships are like the dial lock on a safe. It takes just a few clicks in the right direction – along with some support, accountability, and care – to unlock the door to passion, joy, clarity, confidence, fulfilment, and vitality.

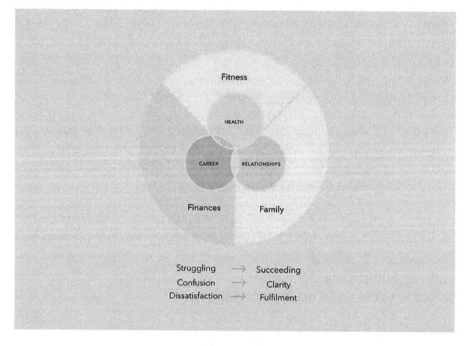

Hell, in my opinion, is never finding your true self and never living your own life or knowing who you are.

-John Bradshaw

▎About the Book

inShape inLove inSpired! is about getting the most you can from this ONE LIFE you have. It is about knowing who you truly are, what sets your soul on fire, and about doing everything you can to ensure your life revolves around those very things.

The three sections of this book are not mutually exclusive. They intertwine and have a relationship with each other. When you lead a life of passion, purpose, and inspiration, you are more likely to be a positive person and, therefore, more likely to take care of your health and fitness.

Similarly, when you look great and feel great as a result of regular exercise and quality nutrition (the topic of section one, inShape), it has a significant effect on your self-esteem, which gives you the confidence to build and nurture positive relationships in your life and leave the relationships that do not benefit you, all of which makes up the topic of the second section, inLove.

You make other self-assured decisions such as ensuring you are in the right career and have adequate levels of faith and belief to get outside your comfort zone and pursue things that set your soul alight, which is the focus of the final section, inSpired.

A large part of this book discusses how to use peak health as the foundation for an abundant life. I take great pride in being a supportive mentor who empowers clients to take responsibility for their health and ultimately their entire life.

If I claim to be an expert in these areas, it is only because I have spent a lifetime studying these topics. I have made every mistake a person can make, and I've come out the other side happier, more fulfilled and more passionate about helping others maximise happiness and fulfilment in their own lives.

The tone is intended to be humorous, raw, real and supportive. At times it may be blunt. The stories and percentages mentioned throughout the book are based on my experiences and anecdotal evidence. This book is designed to help people who may have struggled to get their mindset right to lose weight or to live a life they love. It's not meant to be statistically driven because I want it to be readable.

It's a book for anyone who feels they can squeeze more goodness out of life, but isn't sure where to start or if it's even possible. Taking control of your health and your life is more of a mental battle than a physical one. It can be a sensitive and overwhelming topic at times. There is not a one-size-fits-all approach.

My skill lies in helping you cultivate positive lifestyle changes by guiding you through a process of self-discovery. You will identify the unlimited choices available, enabling you to reach your goals and make them stick. Your own thinking will be challenged.

When you try and make changes you will be questioned by those closest to you. You will learn how to fill your mind with positivity and cultivate the right attitude to promote positive, lasting change. You will discover how you can improve your health in some simple, yet critical ways, making your approach to peak fitness smarter and not harder.

This book is not all about strategy, it is also about mindset and support. I find it is rarely a lack of education that's responsible for someone not being where they want to be with their health and their life in general. I have a strong history of supporting people and walking beside them on the road to improved health, fitness, fulfilment and self-confidence.

I never felt like I fit in growing up, and now I am passionate about creating environments where people feel supported, comfortable, welcome and valued. If I am direct, it is only because I care, and I know there is a better way.

We only have one life and there's no time to muck around. Making progress starts now!

What Others Say About Scott

"I first met Scott in 2001 while I was working at Lend Lease in a dynamic and demanding role. Scott helped me with my own health and well-being and has also worked with Lend Lease as a speaker, trainer and workshop facilitator on the topics of nutrition, exercise, balance and wellness. His content, contribution and delivery style are always well received and the impact of his presence is always immediate. I feel both proud and fortunate to have worked with Scott, both personally and professionally, for almost twenty years. He is an expert in his field."

Yvonne Kostopoulos – Head of Retail, Lend Lease

"I have known Scott for over 18 years and have utilised his services as a health and well-being professional for well over ten years. Scott is the sort of person who makes change - both mental and physical - real. His steady hand, vast knowledge and ongoing accountability have seen me make many positive improvements over the short and long term. These milestones are now very evident in the way I manage my career and my life outside of work. I have observed Scott's ability to work with individuals of all walks of life; from mums and dads, across professional athletes and high-level corporates. His understated style and entrepreneurial flair ensure positive results, with outcomes that become far more reaching than just cosmetic. He gets it."

Troy Phillips – Director, Mortgage Asset Services

"Scott was instrumental in the early years of my career development and the growth of my businesses. I hired him because I saw what he had achieved and it made sense to work with a mentor who walked the talk and was successful in his own right. He helped me transition from a career in the Navy to become a successful business owner. Scott is both scary and insightful! He genuinely wants you to succeed. He packs so much information into every conversation which delights me every time we meet. He takes time to understand my values and each facet of my career and personal life and this has enabled me to launch and operate two successful businesses over a ten-year period while having a great lifestyle along the way. Scott's expertise includes the development of my teams, growth and upskilling of my managers, marketing strategies, customer service and client retention initiatives, increased profitability, cultivating a mindset of success, confidence and abundance, all while focussing on health, relationships and balance."

Wendy Laurence – Health Club Owner

"In 1999, I engaged the services of Scott Capelin as a health coach. At the time, I was an accountant at Ernst and Young, working long hours and suffering from a lack of life balance. Scott's experience and understanding from his corporate background, along with his expertise as a fitness professional, soon enabled me to lose 50 kilograms and see life more clearly. I've known and worked with Scott for the past 20 years and he has been a constant source of knowledge, care and professionalism. His approach is unique in that he has 20 years of experience in business mentoring, leadership, health coaching and lifestyle consulting. He is the complete package and I'd recommend his services to anyone."

Matthew Malouf – Ernst & Young; Wisdom Business Coaching

"My business increased 200% in the time I worked with Scott. I built a national franchise of tutoring centres and was ultimately able to build my business and sell it – all whilst losing ten kilograms and improving my marriage! Scott believes in you, encourages you, educates you and makes you feel like you can do anything! He was a business mentor, health coach and lifestyle consultant all wrapped into one. His approach is both firm and caring and he is an endless source of knowledge and inspiration."

Tina Tower – Begin Bright Early Childhood Learning Centres

"Scott, you have been absolutely priceless on a myriad of levels. You were always the case to beat from the moment we met you. You have been everything you said you would be and even more impressive than I thought you would be. Thank you."

Lisa Harvey – Head of Workplace Experience, AMP

"Throughout my 25-year career in the finance sector, I've seen my fair share of well-being experts – some who made an impact and others who did not. Scott is the standout performer in my eyes, and I dare say his background and experience are both unique and unparalleled. Scott can speak with depth and intelligence on the topics of corporate well-being, relationships, life balance, business, nutrition, spirituality and overall health. He is direct and humorous and adds value to every project he is involved in. He can deliver content through a variety of mediums and always goes the extra mile as a consultant."

Matt Taylor – Associate Director, Capital Markets and Advisory, National Australia Bank

SCOTT CAPELIN

"Every area of my life has improved. After working with Scott, my husband bought me flowers, saying he was so proud of me and my new business and time management skills. I am getting more done in less time, so I can relax with my family more. From the moment I started collaborating with Scott, my work performance improved, I achieved a greater sense of balance in my life and my confidence went through the roof."

Shari Hawkins – Gecko Kids Sports

▌Introduction

People who are struggling can either consciously or subconsciously pull other people down. Think about those closest to you. Do they lift you up, or drag you down? Think about yourself. Do you lift people up, or drag others down?

Do you feel your life has limitless potential, or do you feel stuck?

What can be better than a life of passion, purpose and inspiration?

A life where each day is a blessing? Where you radiate a positive aura and you are an amazing person to be around? Where you are fit, strong, healthy and proud of your appearance? A life where you associate with positive people and cut the energy vampires loose?

A life where you live with a permanent attitude of gratitude; where you see the gift in every situation; where exercise and healthy food choices are fundamental principles of your existence; and where you have things to look forward to?

A life where you maintain a positive attitude and massive levels of mental strength, regardless of what life throws at you? A life where you have a firmly established sense of contentment and conviction with the knowledge you are on the right path?

That's what being **inShape inLove inSpired!** is all about.

Let's take a look at some statistics that are readily available these days:

- Heart disease is the biggest killer in society. One in two people will suffer from heart disease.
- 20% of the population suffer from depression or anxiety.
- One in two men will get cancer. One in three women will get cancer.
- 40% of marriages end in divorce.
- 84% of people do not like their work.
- One in two people are considered to be overweight or obese.

This is NOT NORMAL. Why do we just accept it? How much of this is preventable with awareness, foresight and planning?

So — why are these statistics not alarming people? Why are they not on the news every day? Instead, we hear about a person who was stabbed in their home last night, a sports team who won, what the weather will do tomorrow, a car crash in a dodgy neighbourhood and war in Albania.

Why are we talking about coronavirus and not suicide, obesity, heart disease, cancer and mental health? Ten million people die each year from cancer – that's 30,000 people per day. One person dies every 36 seconds from heart disease. Why do we think paying 40% tax on our gross income and having four weeks off per year, while being nine kilograms overweight is normal? Surely there must be a better way.

Come on … we are better than this! What's going on here? Why are we living like this? I have written this book to keep people from becoming those statistics, and to support people to live lives of great health, abundance and joy.

We were never given the tools to have an amazing marriage. Or to manage money. Or to be a leader. Or to set goals. Or to understand our values. Or to be healthy. In school, I remember asking if we could do a savings and investment plan. The teacher said it wasn't in the curriculum, but we learned how to square dance, play tunnel ball, make music on the recorder and do quadratic equations. They've all come in handy … not. I actually failed the recorder and was belittled by the music teacher. I had to stay after school and practise it. What a waste of time, trying to learn something I had no interest in. I remember sticking my recorder in the exhaust pipe of my music teacher's car and smiling as he drove out of school in a cloud of smoke.

What is your ideal life? Can you write it down? Do you know what it is? Being able to articulate your dream life is the first step. Don't worry about how to make it happen at this stage. In fact, when you start thinking about 'how', that's usually when most people take their dream vision no further because they start thinking logically — which is a passion killer. Ask yourself what your dream life looks like, ask yourself why, then, with a total sense of freedom, write down what your dream day and dream life look like.

Let me tell you about my background, and then I'll let you know more specifically what this book is about.

About Me: Scott Capelin

I am an experienced wellness coach who helps people like you master the areas of health, relationships and living life with passion. My purpose is to maximise the abundance, joy and happiness of those I help, by creating a balance that aligns with their own values.

With a deep understanding of human values, I bring forward the life you want with clarity and focus. I openly reflect on my experiences and the pressure of my own life's challenges after making mistakes with money, life choices, career, and intimacy.

I provide the accountability and tactical support I wish I'd had through the wins and losses, successes and failures in my life. With a business degree and time spent building several businesses in the fitness industry, my education and experience in health and wellness have helped thousands of people unlock the door to a passionate life they love. I take a bird's-eye view of the routines and rituals of my clients, identifying the root causes of struggles, whilst focusing on their individual goals and what's important.

By instilling a philosophy of fantastic health, I help people develop a sense of achievement, along with great vitality, confidence and self-esteem. My clients build a deeply connected relationship with themselves, which translates into loving relationships with others and a life experience that has clarity and meaning. The easy part is working with a client and identifying what needs changing. The hard part is for them to make these changes. But that's where I can help.

As an optimist and futurist, I demonstrate how developing a combination of behaviours that bring one's best self forward, creates opportunities most people only believe are for someone else. It's a practical approach to prioritising time and tasks, making the decisions that allow life to be in alignment with core personal values and building on the success gradually experienced. My approach shares and celebrates the wins, supports and shines a light when it's dark, and transforms the body and mindset.

Now more than ever, everyday people are seeking change in their habits to reduce pain, improve fitness, get better sleep, lose weight, lower stress or simply increase their life span. I aim to be a powerful role model, helping my clients outgrow unhealthy choices, tackle the challenges of social conditioning and develop sustainable lifestyle changes.

I want to help you feel like you're in control. I want you to feel like you can do this. If you've ever felt like it's all a struggle, I want to empower you with your health and with your life.

The Big Three — inShape inLove inSpired!

Why choose these three areas? What do they really refer to? And how do they relate to each other?

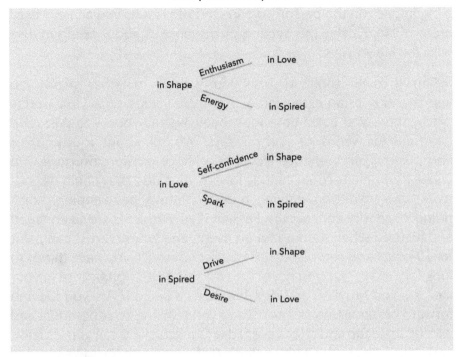

inShape refers to your health. This section covers topics such as exercise, nutrition, and overall health. It discusses food and exercise choices, being at your ideal weight with a body shape you are proud of, and living with mobility, flexibility, energy, and vitality. This is the biggest section of the book and the underlying principle is that peak health is the foundation for a life of abundance. A large part of this section discusses training and nutrition. Over the last 20 years, 95% of my clients have had weight-loss goals. When you become fitter and stronger, and when you maintain your ideal weight, you will feel amazing! Your confidence and self-belief will increase and, from here, you will have a platform to lead a more empowering life.

inLove is about relationships and the influence these relationships have on you, your decisions, your life choices, and your outcomes. This section discusses the relationship you have with yourself, your level of confidence and self-worth, your relationship with your partner, and your relationships with friends, family members, and work colleagues. These relationships are referred to as your 'circle of influence' — the five people you spend the most time with. This has a big impact on the person you are and the results you achieve in all areas of life. Finally, this section of the book is about being in love with the life you live.

inSpired covers topics such as your work — whether or not you love it and if it's an extension of your core values. Or is your work a place where you trade time for money, wait for hours to pass, and hang out for weekends and holidays? We talk about your hobbies and pursuits, and whether you live a life of passion, purpose, and creativity. Pursuits could include raising your kids, they could be your work, travel, knitting, playing music, painting, bee-keeping, horse riding, or charity endeavours. Passion is why athletes are so engaged and focused when training for an event, and why an artist can paint for 10 hours and completely lose track of time. Do you have things to look forward to? Do you have deep meaning and significance in your life? Are you growing and developing as a person? Are you moving forward or remaining stagnant? Are you fulfilling your potential and excited to get up and attack every day? And crucially, can you visualise and articulate exactly what your ideal life looks and feels like?

It's not about the goal. It's about growing to become the person that can accomplish that goal.

- Tony Robbins

The three sections of this book, inShape inLove and inSpired, all have a close relationship with each other. Without having a positive relationship with yourself it's impossible to bring your best self to your relationships with your loved ones. You won't be the best parent or the best partner you can be. If you're not happy, fulfilled, and inspired, you won't be living with maximum energy and vitality. And without great health, you're not going very far at all. Unhappiness leads to poor food decisions and disempowering life decisions which lead to anxiety, stress, depression, unhappiness, poor health, and being overweight. Being overweight leads to eating more, which then leads to lower energy and a negative self-image.

The good news is that starting today, you can make changes – however small – in one or more of these areas. Making a change in one area will flow on to have a positive effect in the other areas. Small changes over time compound to become big changes. Step one to promoting positive change is awareness of what you want and where you want to go. Step two is doing something about it. At the very least, this book is designed to get you thinking. At the very best, it will inspire you to live the life of your dreams. If you're worried about not knowing what you're doing, relax … nobody does! And besides, I'm here to show you how. Let's do it!

▌ Working With Scott

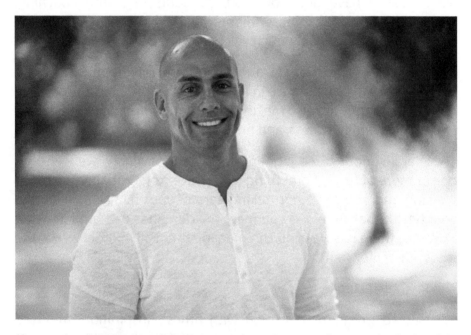

If one doesn't have a life they are passionate about, terrific health, high self-esteem, and a network of supportive relationships around them, it's hard to feel like you're winning.

A life out of balance cannot result in fulfilment. Understanding your values, spending time doing the things you love, building your life around pursuits that light you up, and bringing your best self to your relationships with your loved ones, creates an enormous sense of passion, happiness and confidence. It transforms you into a person you can be proud of.

This is the purpose of my work and what I love helping people achieve. My life's mission is to inspire people to flourish by providing them with the tools and the accountability to embrace their potential so they can experience all the abundance, joy and beauty this life has to offer. My 'Dream Life Design' strategies instil self-confidence in others, by turning confusion into clarity and developing simple and sustainable habits that overcome limiting beliefs.

Since 1999, I have done over 30,000 hours of health coaching, life coaching and business mentoring. I have seen countless transformations, many of which will be outlined in this book.

I am particularly passionate about working with people who are juggling busy lives – they are in relationships, bringing up kids, have careers – and they are also making an effort to improve their health. I refer to it as 'family, fitness, and finances'.

These are like our three juggling balls and inevitably, we will drop one or more of them. Something has to give. You probably can't stop working and you can't stop taking care of your family, so it's often your health that suffers as you meet the demands of a busy lifestyle. However, there is a way you can manage them all in order to get the most out of life.

This is where I step in.

My tailored programs help you with fitness, inspiration, mindset, fulfilment, clarity, confidence and connection in the most important areas of your life. Here's an overview of the different ways you can work with me.

Health and Lifestyle Coaching

Ideal for people who have struggled in the past to maintain an exercise and healthy eating routine. You get me, one-on-one, for a 12-week period where I help you get on track and stay on track.

inShape inLove inSpired!

Wellness Studio Franchising

If you're interested in owning your own business using a proven formula with ongoing support, an inLIFE Wellness franchise might be for you. Check out inlifewellness.com.au

Speaking

If you're looking for an entertaining, knowledgeable, dry, humorous and direct speaker for a conference or event, keynote topics include health, fulfilling potential, and leading a life of passion and inspiration.

Life Coaching

Learn more about yourself in 12 weeks than you have in your entire life. Gain clarity about where you are and where you want to be, set goals and start achieving them.

Women's Weight Loss and Body Shaping Programs

More than a diet and exercise program. Re-educate yourself to maintain a healthier, happier lifestyle.

Business Mentoring

Tailored advice in your areas of need from marketing and finance to managing your team and your mindset. Helpful for both established businesses and people still at the 'ideas' stage.

To learn more about these programs, make an inquiry, or register, please go to www.inlifecoaching.com.au.

All change starts with an intuitive feeling that
there is a better way of being.

- Scott Capelin

If you've had the same recurring thought over
time, it's right, and you have to act on it.

- Scott Capelin

▌ Book Bonus

As a special bonus for reading this book, I would like to offer you free access to my Dream Life Design program.

Dream Life Design is the ultimate process of self-discovery. By completing this course you will learn more about yourself and feel clearer than ever about where you are and where you want to be. Most people go through their whole lives without the kind of clarity and conviction you will gain by working through the exercises included.

The program has 4 modules which are:

MODULE 1: Identify Your Core Values
MODULE 2: Goal Setting
MODULE 3: The End Result
MODULE 4: Plan of Action

You will be guided through the entire process in an efficient and effective manner. By the end you will have:

- Identified your most important personal core values
- Compelling goals set for the next three months, one year, and three year
- Developed a weekly exercise plan
- Created a personalised nutrition strategy
- Created a Dream Board and a Life Vision Statement
- Developed a plan of action to make it all happen!

It's a fun and enlightening process that's designed to take you to a new level in your life!

To access the program go to inlifecoaching.com.au, send a message through the Contact page, and the program will be sent to you!

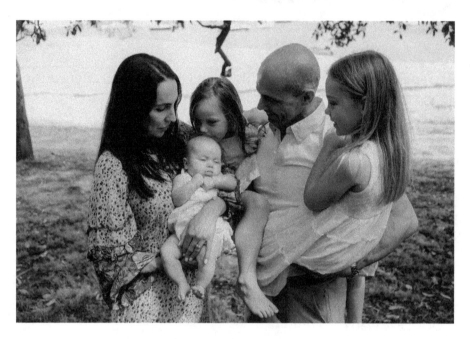

inShape

How To Approach Long-Term Health and Fitness

I have spent over two decades helping people make exercise and healthy eating a regular part of their lifestyle, and have been privileged to be involved with countless life transformations. You can get into the best shape of your life at any age, so let's never use age as an excuse or barrier to becoming healthier and more active.

I love helping people improve their health and vitality, however, it's the flow-on effect that is most interesting. I have yet to meet a person who is in excellent physical shape, and does not feel amazing and get the most out of life. As such, to support you to look and feel your best, we start with getting you into excellent physical shape. This comes down to exercise and nutrition – the subject of this first section of the book.

Many people spend $100 per month on petrol and $150 on Foxtel, yet they won't spend more than $30 per week on health.

Is there anything **more** important to spend money on?

I see people driving a Mercedes with a monthly car repayment of $1,500, but they won't spend $400 a month on personal training.

Decisions regarding how to spend your time, money, energy and headspace come down to your personal values which we cover later in this book. I once had a client who was physically too inflexible to get into his Lamborghini.

A 31-year-old corporate client I worked with has difficulty putting his shoes on in the morning. His tummy got in the way, his joints were immobile and his muscles were weak and inflexible. Working 60 hours per week to have a heart attack at the age of 43 doesn't seem like the right approach for an intelligent, driven person. Living your peak life, at your peak health, starts by looking at your overall well-being and putting long-term daily actions into practice.

The Dalai Lama, when asked what surprised him most about humanity, he said:
"Man. Because he sacrifices his health in order to make money. Then he sacrifices money to recuperate his health. And then he is so anxious about the future that he does not enjoy the present; the result being that he does not live in the present or the future; he lives as if he is never going to die, and then dies having never really lived."

> If your spine is inflexibly stiff at 30,
> you are old; if it is completely
> flexible at 60, you are young.
>
> - Joseph Pilates

What Are 'Urgent' and 'Important' Activities?

In his 1954 speech to the Second Assembly of the World Council of Churches, former U.S. President Dwight D. Eisenhower, quoting Dr. J. Roscoe Miller, President of Northwestern University, said, "I have two kinds of problems: the urgent and the important. The urgent are not important, and the important are never urgent". This 'Eisenhower Principle' is said to be how he organised his workload and priorities.

He recognised that great time management means being effective as well as efficient. In other words, we must spend our time on things that are important, and not just on the things that are urgent. To do this, and to minimise the stress of having too many tight deadlines, we need to understand the distinction between the two.

- Important activities have an outcome that leads to us achieving our goals, whether professional or personal.

- Urgent activities demand immediate attention and are usually associated with achieving someone else's goals. They are often the ones we concentrate on and they demand attention because the consequences of not dealing with them are immediate.

	URGENT	NOT URGENT
IMPORTANT	1. DO	2. PLAN
NOT IMPORTANT	3. DELEGATE	4. ELIMINATE

The thing with health is that many people put it in the 'important, but not urgent' category. Essentially, this means that while people recognise the state of their health is very important, it is not considered urgent to address our health on any given day.

Unlike, for example, paying the electricity bill due that day or replying to a work email about a project due in the next week. The more mundane important tasks often get prioritised over-exercising, getting adequate sleep or eating healthy food. It's easier to put these things off in favour of other pressing tasks.

My stance is that health, or anything you put in the 'important but not urgent' category, is critical to tend to today and every day. If you think of these things as 'not urgent', they will get put off until tomorrow, the next day, the next month or the next year.

The ramifications are not always immediate but will eventually show up. Unfortunately, for many people, they take the form of being 15 kilograms overweight, a heart attack in your 40's or a cancer diagnosis. I want you to consider the idea that plans for exercise and nutrition should be the first thing in your schedule, not the last.

Essential Elements

Sometimes health professionals meet new clients and ask them to change 17 things straight away in order to get fit. A selection of actions they'll dump on their new client include:

- drink more water
- exercise five times per week
- reduce your bread intake
- reduce your dairy intake
- skip breakfast
- eat more protein and natural fats
- do not drink alcohol
- reduce your sugar and gluten intake.

If you're embarking on a fitness journey, being bombarded with all of these mandates is too much. You can become overwhelmed by so many changes and demands, and then you will likely abandon your attempt to get fit.

My approach is to begin with the end in mind and develop a program that is sustainable over the long term while still achieving great results.

For a person to get fit, the plan should happen in manageable stages, bearing in mind the stages aren't one-size-fits-all. Each stage depends on the individual – where they are when they start, how much change they can manage in each stage, and their end goal.

What's the best first stage for you?

How about exercising for 30 minutes, three times a week for one month?

Not right for you?

Maybe two exercise sessions of 20 minutes can be your first stage.

Would that feel like an achievement for you?

Would this plan progress your fitness?

Let's focus on that, and then reassess.

Your first stage: making it about you

I meet lots of people who are looking to establish and maintain a consistent exercise regime after not exercising or eating healthily for at least a few years. It is common to meet people when they are somewhere between five and 15 kilograms overweight, who are at a point where they feel uncomfortable and whose current level of health and fitness is no longer acceptable to them.

Everyone at this point has quite a clear goal — lose that extra weight, feel more comfortable, feel better about yourself and increase fitness. It only takes a few tweaks, in terms of improving exercise and nutrition routines, to see some great results in the short term.

When I meet people wanting to make improvements to their health and fitness, we get their exercise going a little better, and their nutrition going a little better, and they achieve noticeable results straight away. Typically, people experience an increase in energy and feel better immediately after cleaning up their eating habits. Improvements in strength, fitness and energy happen almost immediately with just a small amount of consistent exercise.

Someone who commences an inShape journey begins to experience a lot of positive emotions; they gain a renewed sense of vigour and it becomes an inspirational part of their life. It's pretty amazing to see! The starting stage is absolutely critical and it MUST be a good experience. If you feel like you are achieving something and you CAN do it, success flows from there.

Your next stage: making it fun

The next stage happens three to five months into your inShape journey. At this point, I sometimes wonder if the newfound adherence to exercise will be a three-month fad or something that will be stuck to for the long term.

The critical element for anyone to continue exercising over the course of a year, two years, a decade and a lifetime is whether or not they enjoy it. Is it fun? Enjoying your weekly exercise routine is paramount because it does not matter how good something is for you – if you don't enjoy it, then it probably won't last.

The best exercise routines are the ones when you do activities you enjoy. I repeat: it doesn't matter how good the activity is for you – if you don't enjoy it, then it probably won't last. It should be noted that, broadly speaking, improved health comes down to exercising consistently and eating nutritious food. For most people, the challenging part is eating healthily 24/7/365.

There's a saying that you can't out-train a bad diet, but you can out-train an average one. I see a lot of food diaries that contain pizza, red wine, chocolate, and cheese and crackers, but the owners of these diaries are still losing weight because they are exercising in a consistent and efficient way. Their nutrition might not always be perfect but they manage to be in a calorie deficit most of the time.

I should also note there's a difference between eating for health and eating for weight loss. If your total weekly calorie intake is not excessive, you can include yummy treats in your nutrition strategy every day and still lose weight and end up with the body you want.

Here's a comparison: if you're eating for good health, for breakfast you might have a banana smoothie with spinach, avocado and blueberries, which contains a healthy amount of vitamins and minerals. However, if you're eating for weight loss, that same meal could be inappropriate because it's at the wrong time of the day and it's not an ideal macronutrient composition.

The point to note here is simply that eating to promote good health versus eating to lose weight can be very different. Do you think you're eating well but are frustrated or disappointed with your lack of weight loss? Maybe you're simply eating too much good food, like fruit, for example.

You could be consuming more calories than you're burning, or you could be eating a high-carb, low-fat diet, which has implications for weight gain and loss.

Exercise and healthy eating is a package deal. You eat well, you train well. You train well, you eat well. It is easier to continue doing one if you are doing the other. Healthy and fit people don't wake up and ask themselves if they will exercise that day – they just do because it is part of their lifestyle.

I'll say it again: Exercise and healthy eating is a package deal.

The Four Phases of the inShape Journey

The diagram below illustrates four stages in the journey to being inShape and can be helpful in terms of managing your expectations and understanding wellness needs to be something that lasts long term. This is something I learned with Impact Training and the National Sales Academy when I was in a sales training course, and I think it's very relevant.

1. Initial Phase: the first four weeks. This is when you establish good habits, increase your education, begin your program and start to feel better.
2. Visual Phase: weeks five to eight. It's when you notice results because they show up in your appearance. Others notice these positive changes in your appearance as well.

3. Results Phase: months three to 12. You have achieved your initial goal, such as achieving your desired weight. Please note this can be a dangerous time of regression; it is critical you break through to the next stage! The reason the timeframe here is broad is that it depends on your starting fitness level and the quality of your nutrition and exercise. The reason people often go backwards here is because they have arrived at their goal, and then back off and stop doing the things that saw them get to where they wanted to be.

4. Lifestyle/Maintenance Phase: starts at 12 months and is ongoing. You have maintained your results; exercise and healthy nutrition are part of your lifestyle. Now you have new, more exciting goals.

THE BIG PICTURE

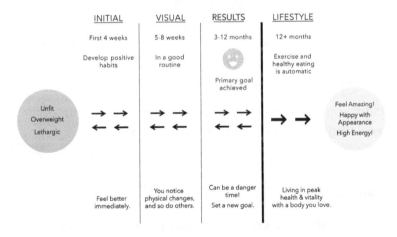

In terms of staying on track over the long term, one of the best philosophies to live by is getting your exercise to be a ten out of ten, and your nutrition to be a seven or eight out of ten. These are scores relating to the quality of each category with ten being the highest quality and one the lowest.

Not many people can get their nutrition perfect, so aiming for seven or higher is still healthy but more realistic and allows for vices such as alcohol, dining out, and some chocolate after dinner. With many people, exercise often ends up being the easy bit and because an ideal health plan is individual, your ten out of ten can be whatever works for you.

Your exercise plan might include taking your dog to the park, doing yoga, swimming laps at the local pool, doing Pilates, aiming for 10,000 steps per day, playing tennis, lifting weights or doing a spin class. It could mean exercising three times per week or eight times per week. Again, it is individual.

It is worthwhile to note that, to achieve the perfect score for the exercise portion of getting healthy, you must place exercise in your diary first and allow everything else to fit around it. Many people place to exercise in their weekly schedule after they've added other commitments.

It doesn't work very well that way. You might think you should get everything else in your personal and professional life done first before you exercise, but the personal and professional to-do list never ends. If you determine when and where your exercise fits, you'll discover you magically get everything else done anyway.

Prioritising your exercise is a key aspect of achieving your goals. It's an issue we'll return to later because it's important.

Expectations

In terms of managing your expectations when you've committed to getting healthy, it is useful to know there will be some sacrifice and an element of deprivation when it comes to food choices, even when you aim for a seven out of ten. It would be nice to think it will be pretty effortless; however, there will be times when you have to say no to chocolate and custard tarts, and you won't like it. Getting back in shape can involve reducing things like alcohol, soft drinks, carbohydrates and your overall calorie intake.

You don't need to be a dietitian to know which foods are good for you and which ones aren't. If you find yourself asking whether or not you should be eating something, the answer is probably no. Sometimes, cutting back your food intake involves a small reduction. Other times, depending on where your health is at and where you want to take it, a major reduction might be necessary.

There will also be times when you don't feel like doing an exercise session or you are pushed for time. Recently, an older gentleman said to me, "If I only ever exercised when I felt like it, I would never exercise". I thought this was a good point.

Personally, I love to exercise. However, I would estimate that around 50% of the time, when I am scheduled to do a training session, I don't feel like it. I can always think of 25 other things I could be doing instead. Those other things will still be there in 45 minutes, but the problem with missing an exercise session is that we cannot go back and do 'today' again. To achieve results, we must make consistent exercise a priority.

One more thing – please schedule exercise at a time when it's not going to be interrupted by work and family commitments. As tough as it sounds, this could mean exercising at 5:30am.

Why?

There's a much greater chance of the day getting away from you, if you're a busy person trying to exercise at 5pm.

I have a friend who used to own a car dealership. He told me that for years he had customers who would buy a car using finance, and then return at some stage and trade the car in to upgrade. Often, when trade-in time came, the car was not worth as much as the finance owing, so they added the difference to the new car loan. This would happen multiple times, and my friend explained that, at some point, the purchaser has to 'own it', meaning they have to pay off the finance that's been accruing over previous years.

This hurts. I think about getting in shape the same way. If you have been out of shape for five, ten or 20 years, you've had your fun and it's time to own it. I do have a signature approach to exercise and nutrition that I believe is about as effortless as it can get.

However, lifestyle shifts can be tough. Banana bread is nice, but it isn't going to help you lose weight. Say no to it and deal with it. Ask yourself if you would prefer eating banana bread for 5 minutes, or being happy with your body 24/7.

If you have been out of shape for 20 years, you won't fix it in three months. Get used to saying no for a while, especially when making food decisions. Every positive decision adds up. Consider every compulsion, urge or craving to be like a fork in the road.

Habit says to eat it. Discipline says no.

The more times you make a healthy choice, the fitter you get, step by step. A large part of my work involves assisting intelligent, lovely people who know what to do but are not doing it. What I repeat to them, and what they soon experience themselves, is: every positive resolution you make is a step forward.

Unfortunately, positive decisions relating to food usually involve saying no to something. That's the reality, especially at the beginning.

It's important to note that the only way to lose weight and also eat junk food is if you find a way to remain in a calorie deficit. This means burning more calories than you eat. It can be achieved. It's called flexible dieting or IIFYM (If It Fits Your Macros). While I don't advocate this kind of eating plan, it does exist. It's basic common sense to know that everything is okay in moderation.

The problem with moderation is that many people eat lots of things in moderation. They have some toast and peanut butter in moderation, cappuccinos in moderation, a glass of wine and some chocolate in moderation – all on the same day, every day. It adds up.

Your ability to successfully get fit and healthy largely depends on your ability to delay gratification in the moment. Eating foods you know are bad for you could be referred to as self-sabotage. People tell themselves they can always start tomorrow. Or next Monday. Or in January. Five years later, it's still happening. So, get used to being hungry. Go to bed peckish. When you're hungry, quieten the stomach with a snack or drink. Not a large meal.

Delayed gratification is only hard at that moment. Be strong! There is no magic fix. You'll feel like you're depriving yourself, but it passes in 60 seconds. Move on – you'll be proud you did. It will become a habit, then a routine. Small changes over time add up and become big changes.

Ideally, the fulfilment you derive from making better food choices, exercising regularly and improving the shape of your body will result in feelings of achievement that totally outweigh the negatives associated with knocking back a bit of junk food.

**It is in your moments of decision
that your destiny is shaped.**

- Tony Robbins

Most of the time, when I meet a new client they are ready to make a change. In our initial consultation, we cover goals such as weight loss, increasing strength and fitness, and being consistent with exercise.

That's all fair enough but the true goal runs much deeper. If you were to ask someone why they had these goals, they might say something like, "So I can look good at the beach" or "So I can fit into my old clothes".

If we were to probe a little further, the deeper reason always comes back to emotion: to become more confident, more proud of my appearance, to be happier. Losing ten kilograms and being able to do 30 push-ups is one thing; however, the most exciting part is the way improved health, wellness and body shape makes you feel emotionally.

In the following chapters, I'll show you how to make your overall approach to getting inShape simpler, smarter, more efficient, personal and realistic – all while achieving better results and ultimately becoming happier and having a more positive self-image.

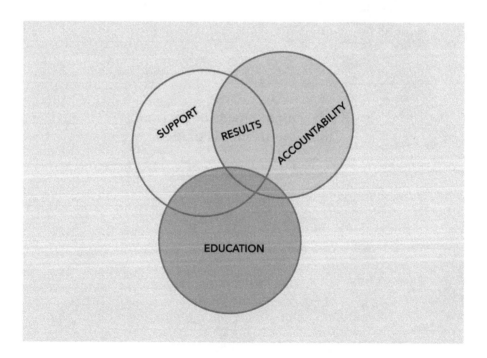

What Is Your WHY for Peak Health?

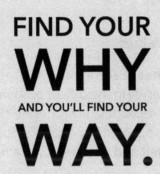

FIND YOUR
WHY
AND YOU'LL FIND YOUR
WAY.

- John C. Maxwell

We all know we should exercise and eat healthy foods, so why do we sometimes treat exercise like it's optional?

Why do we consciously purchase a block of chocolate, take it home, eat all of it and then feel guilty?

If we would prefer to be healthy and in good shape, rather than carrying a spare tyre around our mid-section, why won't we just make changes to our lifestyle?

Well, there are a few answers to this question, and the psychology behind sabotaging behaviour runs deep, however, one reason is that we haven't identified and connected to our 'Why?'

For most of us, exercise and healthy nutrition choices don't come naturally or easily.

So, what do we do?

What could motivate or inspire us to put in the effort and reach our peak health if it doesn't come naturally?

The aim of this chapter is to help you identify the most influential reasons 'why' and encourage you to put in the effort to achieve your health goals.

Standards and Core Values

How often have you heard someone (yourself) say: "I can't help it. There's always a jar of candy in the office," or "I was at a work conference and I had to eat the croissants". Is someone threatening you to eat these things; leaving you with no choice? How about: "Well, I can't cook one meal for myself and another for the rest of the family".

Actually, you could – or your family could eat what you eat, or make their own. The best results come when you take ownership of your behaviours, actions, and outcomes, and when you see how your small daily choices are linked to your health and weight.

Ultimately, it comes down to identifying your inspiration behind wanting to be in top shape and then connecting with it on a deep level.

Values and standards are closely related. When I'm being nice, I say, "It's okay, perhaps you're not performing well in this particular area of your life because it's not high on your hierarchy of personal core values".

When I'm being firm, I ask my clients to assess their personal standards:

"Do you feel that you have high standards for your health, your work, and the quality of your life?

Or are you settling for something less than you know you can achieve?"

Do low standards in an area indicate low values? You could place a high value on being in great shape but still, have low standards. For example, you might want to be healthy, but you eat junk food every day. You may place low value on having a good social life but still have high standards in that area.

The following diagram shows the relationship between values and standards.

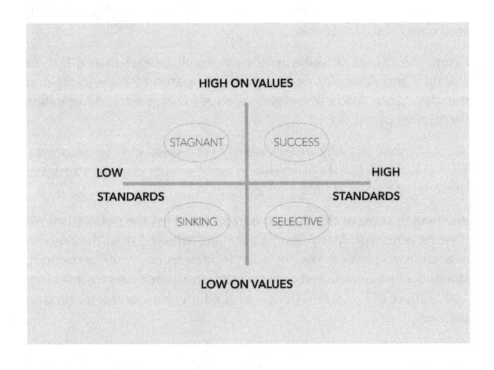

In summary, from this diagram:

- Low standards and high values: you won't get anywhere
- Low standards and low values: you'll go backwards fast
- Low values and high standards: you'll achieve something ... maybe, sporadically, slowly
- High values and high standards: you'll win

Stress

Stress results in weight gain. It prevents weight loss. It increases the production of stress hormones, such as cortisol. It leads to inflammation. Inflammation causes weight gain. Weight gain leads to increased inflammation. It's a nasty cycle. I meet a lot of people with sore knees and a bad back.

Often, the causes of these issues are much deeper than a lack of strength and flexibility, or any problem related to their joints and muscles. Stress leads to emotional issues that eventually manifest themselves physically.

We can't figure out why we lack energy, can't sleep, are in pain, or why we feel bloated, but it's often due to emotional or physical stress. We think being busy and time-poor is normal.

We think the cost of city-living is normal. We think the polluted air we breathe is normal. Many people are more stressed than they realise or acknowledge. We make our worst food decisions when we're tired, stressed, emotional, bored or depressed, and quite often we're feeling one or more of these emotions – all the time! No wonder it's hard to eat well.

I have two colleagues who are experts in the field of Chinese medicine. They say that stress produces toxic hormones that accumulate around your stomach area, and to protect us, our body shrouds these toxins in body fat so they cannot leak into our bloodstream.

Isn't that fascinating?

I meet quite a few people wanting to lose weight. Their exercise regime is consistent and their nutrition habits are pretty good, however, they are highly stressed and the scales don't budge.

Chinese medicine practitioners say we have too much Yang in our lives and we need to balance it out with more Yin. They say that rather than exercising harder, which can further increase the production of stress hormones, some people are better off doing yoga, having a rest, taking a bath, reading a book, or sitting in a chair for 20 minutes doing some breathing exercises.

To explain this, these Chinese Medicine practitioners tightly clasp their hands and say this is an analogy for our muscle cells. When we are stressed, the body holds tightly to fat and everything is so tense we can't release anything.

The solution is to relax and chill out.

Easier said than done? Maybe.

But many people in the western world would certainly benefit from some kind of lifestyle change, rather than a quick fix.

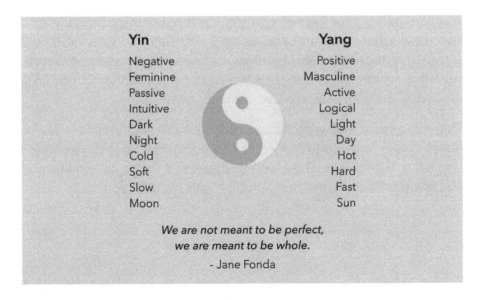

Yin	Yang
Negative	Positive
Feminine	Masculine
Passive	Active
Intuitive	Logical
Dark	Light
Night	Day
Cold	Hot
Soft	Hard
Slow	Fast
Moon	Sun

*We are not meant to be perfect,
we are meant to be whole.*

- Jane Fonda

Seeing a naturopath can help with weight loss. A naturopath can do a simple saliva test and determine what's happening internally with key hormones such as cortisol, estrogen and progesterone. They may also tell you that we don't rest enough these days, and we spend a lot of time stressed which puts our system in a "fight or flight" response.

When this is the case, the digestive function does not happen optimally. You could reset your system with a detox or cleanse, increase the amount of fibre and nutrients in your diet, and improve your gut microbiome.

You might go to a chiropractor, kinesiologist or homeopath and through a few simple tests learn that your adrenal glands are running on empty, or your liver or kidneys aren't functioning normally, or you're low in iron. You might go to the GP and get a referral for a blood test and discover you're insulin resistant or your thyroid isn't performing the way it should.

When it comes to health, and in particular weight loss, or even other factors such as skin conditions or poor sleep, there are the external, controllable factors that are visible and controllable such as what we eat and how much exercise we do, and there are the internal, unseen factors that we may not be aware of, and don't know how to optimise.

You can't tell if your liver or kidneys are functioning optimally, or if you have a hormonal imbalance, or if you have adrenal fatigue. If something doesn't feel right and you can't identify the issue it's worth seeing a variety of health and wellness professionals to obtain a diagnosis. Without assessing, you're just guessing.

There can be a few ways to approach health and wellness and it doesn't have to be complicated or confusing. You never know which approach will unlock the door to increased levels of vitality and abundance. Go with an approach that feels right for you.

Motivation and Inspiration

Inspiration is not the same as motivation. The two are not synonymous. Motivation is when you have a goal, but you need to constantly fire yourself up, or have someone fire you up, to drive yourself towards an outcome. Imagine physically grabbing your goal and dragging it over hot coals until you get to where you want to be. That can be okay, but typically it's hard work – and hard work is usually not sustainable over the long term. Reaching peak health and maintaining it requires something more than motivation.

You need inspiration. Inspiration is when the goal propels you. It's when the outcome is such an intrinsic part of who you are, that you cannot live without the attainment of your desire. This is a much better headspace to be in than what motivation provides.

The way to find the inspiration to support yourself in meeting your goals involves connecting your peak health to your top values. It helps when you link 'being in shape' to the things in your life that you most value.

For example, you might not love exercising or eating salad, but if you're a parent, doesn't it make sense to be the fittest, most positive parent you can be?

Here, you would link 'getting into peak health' with your children. You understand exactly how the two are connected and use that connection to inspire you to exercise and eat well every day.

Consider this: are you a role model to your kids because you make time to exercise, take time for yourself, surround yourself with positive relationships, and make healthy food choices?

Of course, you want to be, but are you?

If you're overweight and cranky on a regular basis is this a positive role model for your kids?

No parent wants to be a negative role model, but be honest with yourself – what are you modelling?

Do you want to see your grandchildren well into their 30s and 40s?

Do you want to be a young 65-year-old or an old 45-year-old?

The point is – you can use your highest value, in this case, your children and grandchildren, and link it to getting into peak health, giving you the necessary inspiration to achieve your health goals.

Another top value to link to is the kind of aging you'd like to experience. After all, it's not all about the number of years in your life, it's about the life in those years. You could be a decrepit 40-year-old or an energetic 85-year-old with loads of energy and a wicked sense of humour.

I meet people in their 30s, 40s, 50s and 60s, who live in pain and are so immobile that they take six minutes to get out of bed in the morning. This stuff doesn't fix itself – you have to do something about it!

And again, if you won't do it for yourself, link it back to your family – can you do it for your kids or grandkids?

Are you setting a good example for your loved ones with your health, your food choices, your relationship choices and your career choices?

Another top value that people have is the work they do.

As such, you could link peak health to this top value. What do you do for work?

Is it leaving a legacy you will be proud of?

Or are you going to say that you don't have the luxury of choice?

If your career is the most important part of your life, do you think you would do better at work if you have mental clarity and are jumping out of your skin with energy and creativity?

If you value mental acuity, you could link it to peak health.

How?

Your brain functions much better after you exercise, and you're much sharper mentally when you undertake intermittent fasting (see the Weight Loss and Nutrition chapter for an explanation).

This link to mental acuity then becomes a deeply inspiring way to engage with exercise and good nutrition on a daily basis.

One of my long-term clients, Yvonne, is a senior executive at Lend Lease. On Mondays and Fridays, she exercises early in the morning and then goes to the office. Her team says that these are her 'ideas days' –when she's on fire with resourcefulness and imagination.

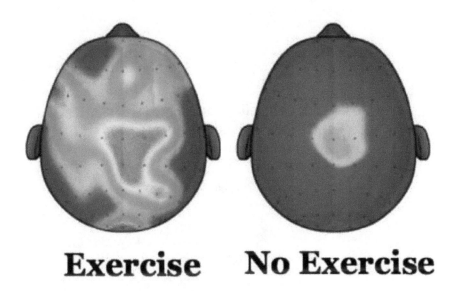

Exercise   No Exercise

If you don't have great reasons to live in your best physical shape, it's hard to be inspired to do so for the long term. The inspiration to put in long-term effort to achieve and maintain peak health comes from linking it to the things you most value in life, for example, your children and family, your experience of aging, your work, your passions and pursuits such as travel, or your mental sharpness.

Another long-term client of mine is a woman called Patsy. She is in her 80's and looks at the world with extreme gratitude and childlike wonder. She exercises every week and travels the world every year with a group of retirees. She says that when they do bus tours throughout Europe and South America, stopping at the amazing tourist destinations on the planet, she and her husband are the only ones who get off the bus. Everyone else is too unfit, weak and lethargic to get out amongst it.

Above all else, you just have to do it for yourself. Nobody else. You have to want to do it for yourself. No other form of extrinsic motivation will last.

> **To keep the body in good health is a duty, otherwise we shall not be able to keep our mind strong and clear.**
>
> - Buddha.

Your Optimal Well-Being

'Wellness' and 'well-being' are broad terms, and it's worth thinking about what they mean to you.

Can you relate to any of the following, in terms of what optimal well-being means to you?

- Living at your ideal weight
- Being fit, healthy and energetic
- Being surrounded by people who love and care for you, and who you love and care for in return
- Having a great social life
- Travelling the world

- Doing work you love
- Having a purpose greater than yourself
- Having hobbies, pursuits, passions and interests in your life
- Having things to look forward to
- Being optimistic and having a positive attitude
- Living with a sense of fulfilment
- Maintaining a high degree of self-confidence
- Having a rewarding intimate relationship
- Liking the home you live in
- Enjoying your work
- Giving and receiving praise and recognition
- Having an element of creativity and adventure in your life
- Having a sense of spirituality
- Feeling like your work-life balance is in order
- Feeling like you are growing, learning, developing and progressing in some way, on a constant basis
- Being happy with the way you look
- Feeling like you have autonomy and control in your life
- Being in a good financial position
- Having a sense of community and connection in your life

It could be argued that most of these points have something to do with well-being and living your best life. However, everyone looks at the world differently, and some of these areas will inevitably be more or less important to each person. The point is that if you value many or any of the above, then you value your well-being. You can then harness that to inspire yourself to put in the daily effort to reach or maintain peak health.

Long-Term Peak Health

People often say to me, "Send me a food plan". What they mean is they want me to write out exactly what they should and should not eat for every meal, every day. I am not a proponent of food plans. In fact, I grew disillusioned with them a long time ago, when I knew I was spending time writing out food plans for people I knew weren't going to follow them. It's not that they were lazy or undisciplined. It's just not feasible to follow a food plan long term. Inevitably, we go off the plan. We might be out at a restaurant, or we are at home and just not prepared with the planned food. Nobody follows a diet long term.

Writing food plans for people can help as a guide and for some inspiration, however, it's not realistic to eat the same thing long term. I think what helps most people is ideas, tips, tricks, education, and providing a framework that offers some flexibility.

The best solution by far is finding out what works for you, and figuring it out for yourself. You can do it. Try different things, ask yourself how you feel when you eat certain foods or eat a certain way.

Are you happy with your weight and how you look and feel?

If not, try something else. You don't need someone else to tell you how to eat or what to eat. It's funny that human beings are by far the smartest animals on the planet yet half the time we aren't sure how to feed ourselves. You won't see a tiger roaming the plains of Africa turning around one day saying "That's it guys, I'm going vegan".

When developing a nutrition strategy, there's a set of criteria it must meet to maximise the chances of success. The plan I develop for someone must be:

- simple
- flexible
- practical
- enjoyable
- personal
- effective

In fact, it is not about being on a diet, it's about an achievable approach to nutrition and exercise, designed to achieve extraordinary results.

Learn to cook and prepare food, even if it's just a few key meals. Write your own food plan. Buy the food and prepare it. Have some healthy pre-prepared meals in the fridge, ready to go. There are some terrific brands out there now that make ready-to-eat meals. It's not hard to be healthy in a convenient and cost-effective way.

Learn how to make chia pudding, Brussels sprouts and bacon, green smoothies, and lamb cutlets with broccoli and corn. Drink two litres of water per day. Have a protein shake instead of a meal if you have nothing prepared.

Don't blame your partner or the kids because the food in your home isn't perfect for you. You also don't have to eat poorly on the weekend or go crazy at the social gathering on Friday night.

I encourage doing forms of exercise that you prefer and enjoy, with consistency and high frequency if possible, in a way that is low on impact and moderate in intensity.

The Power of Compelling Goals

Most of us want to look great and live with optimal health, but don't always do what needs to be done to get there. I have worked with many people, in a health-coaching capacity, who did not achieve any significant results for a long period of time until they developed a more compelling goal. People often want to be like the healthy, fit people they see but aren't prepared to do what they do.

Here are some examples of clients who didn't make health gains until they had a compelling goal:

Louise didn't lose any weight for two years. She felt it was a hormonal issue when, in fact, she was eating too many cookies and snack foods. Then she became engaged to her boyfriend and the wedding was booked for ten months later. Louise lost 12 kilograms between her engagement and the wedding.

What this shows is that without a compelling goal, in this case, her wedding, Louise wasn't inspired to make the needed changes in her behaviour that would enable her to lose weight. Once she had that goal, however, she made those changes and achieved the success she sought.

Tim was 26 years old and 115 kilograms. He was always the larger-than-life 'big man'. It became his identity although you could see it didn't sit comfortably with him. Tim was made redundant from his job and he wanted to join the fire department.

He had to pass the fitness test and lose 15 kilograms. He lost 22 kilograms and has enjoyed a fruitful career as a fireman for the last nine years. Again, once Tim had a compelling goal, he was inspired to make the changes he'd been yearning to make for years, but hadn't. It didn't stop there though. Tim achieved his initial goal and set more goals. He is now very passionate about triathlons and enters them regularly.

Troy, 51 years old, was always fit and strong. He exercised regularly, although his weight was always over 130 kilograms. His best friend suffered a serious health issue and passed away.

After this, Troy's mindset shifted. He stopped drinking alcohol, took up intermittent fasting, had a comprehensive series of health tests, and lost 35 kilograms. It seemed the death of his best friend was the tragic, but inspiring, deep push Troy needed to get healthy.

Action Item

Take a moment to have a think about what the process of becoming the healthiest you can be would look like. Take note of the word 'process'. It's not the outcome.

Grab a pen and paper, or use the Notes app on your phone, and stop for a minute to outline exactly what you would do for exercise, what you would do with your nutrition, and what else you would add to your week or month to increase your level of self-care.

> **The first step in creating optimal health
> is to know your "why".
> Why do you want to be healthy?
> My why is simple. I want to be full of energy, focus,
> and strength to live fully everyday and do
> whatever I want without restriction.**
>
> - Dr. Mark Hyman

In a perfect world, what would your optimal well-being regimen look like? Use your imagination and have some fun with it, and forget limitations such as time, money and who will look after the kids.

- Would you walk four times a week, take up yoga, do five classes a week at the gym, have a monthly massage, or see a chiropractor every quarter for optimal spine health?
- Would you do a flexibility class once per week or a morning fast three days per week?
- Would you do a juice detox, have a colonic, or book yourself into a health retreat once a year with a friend?
- Would you have organic food home-delivered once a week?
- Would you take up Pilates, meditation, strength training or swimming?

The best exercise plans are the ones you enjoy, so make sure you include things you will look forward to.

Most importantly, be clear about your reason for doing it all. Ideally, you would do it for YOU. Not to impress anyone else. Exercise does not always have to be about weight loss and getting fitter.

It is often a mental outlet, or the only time you can get an hour to yourself when you're not parenting or working.

Exercise is a time when you are not at home, you are not at work, and you get to do something that is just for you — this time is sacred and it should be highly valued and respected!

Do you have to be selfish sometimes to get your exercise in? Hell, yes! And, if you know why you're doing this, then it's nothing to be ashamed of.

Accountability Makes Everything Happen Faster

> **Accountability is the glue that bonds commitments to results.**
>
> - Will Craig

I spend most of my time working with extremely nice people who are intelligent and successful. However, when it comes to their exercise and nutrition, they know what they should be doing but they aren't doing it. Education isn't always the issue.

The issue is often accountability – the theme of this chapter.

Back in 2007, I had a business coach. One day, in passing, he said, "Accountability makes everything happen faster". I reflected on this and realised he was right. To take it one step further, accountability is often the difference between making something happen, and it not happening at all.

Jordan Peterson has a best-selling book called *12 Rules for Life*. One of his rules is: "Treat yourself like you are someone you are responsible for". People treat their children, and often their pets, better than they treat themselves. You might let yourself down but you will usually have too much integrity to let someone else down. This is how a good coaching or mentoring relationship works, and this is where the power of accountability lies.

I have a financial advisor, a business mentor and a life coach. I don't have these people because I don't know what to do. I know what to do – it's just that, sometimes, I don't do it. The accountability of answering to someone makes me do it; plus, it's fun having a sounding board and working with people I like and respect, who are where I want to be in certain areas of my life. It's also inspiring to aim to be continually improving. I believe, in life, you are either growing or you are dying.

Sometimes I simply get confused, and I want to ensure I make the right decisions and stay on track, so it's great having these people available. Great coaches can see things much more clearly than we can. They are external, objective and have the skills to ask the right questions which, in turn, enable us to ask and answer questions for ourselves. Ownership of your decisions is where the true power lies, rather than being simply told what to do.

The process of writing this book has been enormous. It's something I have wanted to do for years, so I sought out a way – accountability – to make sure I did it and did it well. To establish this accountability, I paid the publisher and editor, agreed on a timeline, met the deadlines, and you're looking at the end result.

Without that accountability, this book would still just be an idea bouncing around inside my head. People will let themselves down but they won't let someone else down, especially if there's a ramification for doing so.

Your Health and Fitness Accountability

When it comes to health and fitness, you really don't have to do it alone. You can and should establish a system of accountability there, too. There are so many people who can help if you need nutrition assistance, or guidance to help you be consistent and stay on track with exercise.

With most of my clients, we do measurements each week. With this regular check-in, it isn't about what nutrition plan you are following, it's knowing you will have your measurements taken every Friday that ensures you make the right food and exercise choices during the week.

In this way, accountability is established, and it acts as part of their inspiration to make positive choices during the week.

On the topic of accountability, some people need a cuddle, while others need a kick up the butt, to inspire them to make appropriate health choices and achieve their goal of peak health. One of my long-term clients is an elderly lady who says, "There is the carrot and the stick".

The carrot is the goal we strive towards.

The stick is what you get when your behaviour is not in line with your goals. 95% of the time, support and encouragement work better than being firm or getting stern with someone. For this reason, I believe exercise should be a bright part of your day and a positive part of your life – not a 'kick up the butt'.

Some days, just making it to the gym or going for a 20-minute walk might be the very best you can do – without having to worry about setting records when you get there. You don't need more stress added to your week by getting grilled about what you have or haven't eaten, or why you were two minutes late. Like any good relationship, a coach/client partnership works well when it is based on trust, respect and open communication.

The trainer is supposed to provide the motivation; however, the trainer needs to be motivated too. A trainer's motivation matches the client's desire. If it is clear the client isn't doing their part, it's hard for a trainer to care long-term. Sometimes I say to people, "Don't make me do this just for the money".

There has to be a deeper reason and a feeling of fulfilment associated with the constant ongoing progress. This is true for the client as well as the trainer.

A fitness industry survey once revealed that if people join a gym and receive no support, they are likely to be in the same shape, or even worse, after six months. The three reasons given for this outcome were:

- lack of exercise frequency
- lack of education and accountability
- lack of intensity in training.

The best thing about hiring a professional to walk alongside you on your health and fitness journey is these three issues are resolved immediately. In my experience, the likelihood of success increases immensely when you have the assistance of a trainer or coach.

A fitness professional can wear many hats – nutritionist, exercise programmer, trainer, friend, disciplinarian, psychologist and counsellor. A health coach is your cheerleader and supporter in your pursuit of peak health.

There will be ups and downs. You don't have to be perfect. You can still enjoy the foods you love. That's where morning fasting can be the ultimate compensation strategy. (More on that later.)

If you do something that's not perfect, you are not a failure. Start again with the next meal or the next training session. Our aim is to create momentum and be exercising and eating well daily – most of the time.

The focus should be on creating a trend of improvement over the next three to six months. Seeing progress provides the inspiration to want to keep going and to keep improving.

Improvements won't be linear. You will lose weight some weeks and stay the same other weeks. You'll lose, then hold steady. Increase, decrease and hold. Some weeks you will exercise six times and some weeks twice might be all you can manage.

Over time, when you have been consistent with your exercise and nutrition, losing an average of 300 grams per week, before you know it, you'll have lost ten kilograms in eight months and you'll look and feel better than you have in 20 years. Regular accountability for most people is critical.

The concept of accountability does not only apply to health and fitness. Many times over the years, I have walked an extremely fine line between health coaching and life coaching. In the goal-setting process, my clients have committed to broader goals, such as leaving jobs they dislike, moving on from unfulfilling relationships, and even saving money.

Having someone who cares and sticks with you on the path to a better life, greatly increases the chances of you evolving as a person. An accountability partnership really is that powerful.

Sometimes it can be tough, especially at the start, but as an author and spiritual teacher, Robin Sharma says, "Change is hard at first, messy in the middle, and gorgeous at the end".

It is through accountability to another person or group of people that each of us sticks it out to reach that 'gorgeous end'.

To begin, begin.

William Wordsworth

Above and Below the Line

The diagram below is a powerful model for behaviour and mindset change. It was first presented to me in 2006 when I hired my first business coach with a company called Action International. People who succeed in life take ownership and responsibility for their actions, behaviour and results, and they also seek accountability.

People who don't do so, will blame others, make excuses, live in denial, and try to justify the reasons for their lack of progress. Our aim is to live above the line.

It's not about never blaming anyone or anything again. It's about catching yourself when you're making excuses and realising that at the core of it all is you, and if you want something, you can find a way to do it.

Above the line:

1.) Ownership
2.) Accountability
3.) Responsibility

Below the line:

1.) Blame
2.) Excuses
3.) Denial

VICTORS

VICTIMS

Support

I derive a great deal of fulfilment through developing positive relationships with clients and helping them on the path to improved health and fitness. I sincerely believe that 'support and accountability' is the difference between success and failure. I have a spiritual belief that it is our duty to support people if we have the skillset they need.

I also have a belief that all the support we need is available to us, and quite often we think it isn't. All we have to do is seek it out and ask, and what you'll find is that people are happy to help.

I love helping people change the way they look at their wellness and how they look at their life — and to help them make changes over the long term. Sometimes results happen fast and sometimes they happen slowly, but when you look back over a period of six to 12 months of small positive steps forward, the results are enormous.

I GET BY
with a little help
FROM MY FRIENDS

-John Lennon

Incremental steps, better habits and tiny, consistent positive changes lead to significant improvements in the medium and long term.

The best approach I have found to assist people is through support, combined with education and weekly accountability. Checking in with someone who cares and supports you and who will keep you on track and challenge you when you are not doing your best will help you attain your goals.

The support is often about meal ideas, calories, and exercise programs. However, more often than not, it's about journeying with someone and knowing that while they might sometimes let themselves down, they won't let someone else down.

Support is the theme of my life. I have received a lot, and I like to give a lot. I am here to serve. Some people think service is beneath them; however, in many cultures, serving others is the noblest way to live. Support can be as simple (and effective) as checking in on someone and asking how they are.

A good coaching relationship isn't magic. It's a lot more subtle than that. It's a partnership built on trust and understanding. It's a series of conversations and mind shifts over an extended period of time. It's facilitating the shift in a client's mindset to make better decisions.

It is also the accountability of knowing you will be checking in each week that leads to better decisions. In a great client/coach relationship, the coach often believes in the client, and what they can achieve, more than the client does.

The client knows the coach cares and believes in them, and self-belief increases as a result of this. Better decisions are made which lead to better outcomes, momentum builds, and lives are transformed.

I really believe in the power of support and accountability from someone who is on your team — be it a business coach, counsellor, life coach, financial advisor, sports coach, dietitian or friend. Support can be the difference between massive success and going backwards or nowhere.

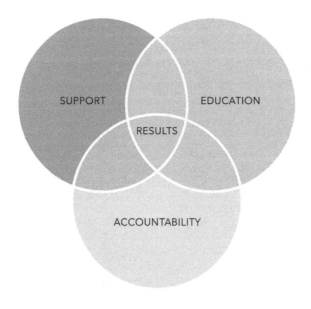

There has to be a line in the relationship. Many professional relationships fall down and lose effectiveness because they become too familiar over time.

We cannot just be friends. You rely on me to help you with a specific set of goals, so let's both pull our weight and get there together.

Anyone who ever achieved anything worthwhile probably didn't do it alone.

▌ Weight Loss and Nutrition

Over the years, I have had thousands of people come to see me, wanting to improve their health and fitness. We start with a consultation, talking about their exercise history, lifestyle, and injuries or medical considerations. We take measurements. And then we discuss goals.

In the majority of cases, weight loss is the goal, and people are keen to discuss their exercise plan. However, since nutrition is the more important component when it comes to weight loss, we end us discussing food for the next half-hour.

I still hear people say, "I am killing myself with exercise and the weight isn't coming off".

I just want to say, "Let's take a look at your diet".

As a matter of fact, the harder people train, the more their appetite increases, making the nutrition bit even harder! Sometimes, I see a person laboriously road-running, looking like they are hating life.

I just want to pull my car over and talk to them about what they are eating.

Before this chapter begins, I'd like to say that I meet many people who want to make positive changes, which should be applauded. I feel like I catch people at an easy time because they have already made the decision to change, and sometimes that decision takes years to make.

Conversations often start with what people are unhappy with and what they feel uncomfortable about, and a plan is developed to make improvements. I believe you should not spend all your time focusing on what you feel is wrong with your health and your body.

There's a good chance that you have two arms and two legs that function, and you have eyes that can read this, and you have the ability to exercise and make choices, and go outside and enjoy the sunshine, and you live in a free society.

There are so many positives right under our nose and it only takes a moment to acknowledge them and instantly you can feel better. I suppose what I'm trying to say is that it's good for the soul to focus on the things that are going well, rather than dwell on what is not optimal. And there are so many things that we can appreciate right now!

Ok, so now let's get into the nitty-gritty…

When it comes to nutrition, it's not one-size-fits-all. It can be really different for individuals, based upon:

- likes and dislikes
- upbringing
- religion
- lifestyle (work hours, young kids, travel)
- humanitarian reasons
- vices (sweet foods, savoury foods, alcohol, soft drinks, lollies/candy, carbs, fast food, chocolate)
- things you read on the internet
- how different styles of eating make you feel.

I like to help people develop a style of eating that is:

- simple
- flexible
- practical

- enjoyable
- personal
- effective

Meeting these criteria increases the likelihood of people sticking with the plan from the outset and making it sustainable. Sometimes, it takes some back and forth, a few conversations, and even a few different nutrition strategies to get this right.

I always say that working with a personal trainer or health coach should not just be a physical experience, it should be an educational one.

For every individual, I believe there's a key that unlocks the door to massive results. Sometimes, we immediately find the key that fits. Other times, it takes a while and some experimentation to find the right approach. It is not one-size-fits-all. The main consideration is not even just the approach to exercise and nutrition – there are emotional factors and lifestyle considerations that result in many different ways to tailor an approach to meet the six criteria above.

A client may work with a health coach for three months, learn new things, implement them and then benefit from the experience for the next 20 years.

When working with a client, I do the following:

- Develop a plan
- Implement the plan
- Measure and monitor the results of the plan
- Change things where necessary

Food plans can sometimes get a bit fancy, detailed, confusing and complicated. Instead, simply remember the basics, eat light, and minimise the consumption of fast food, bread, dessert, biscuits, chocolate, ice cream and alcohol.

A lot of people achieve amazing results by having a coffee or two in the morning, a protein and salad-based lunch, an optional afternoon snack and a healthy dinner.

Eating two to three medium-sized meals each day achieves the goal of creating a calorie deficit, allows for fat loss, and is extremely powerful when combined with the optimal type and frequency of resistance training and overall weekly exercise. It's also a very simple strategy to implement. Most people underestimate how many calories they consume in a day or a week, and overestimate how many calories they burn.

I speak a lot about nutrition because it is mostly responsible for fat loss. In a moment, I will explain the difference between 'fat loss' and 'weight loss'.

Some people say that losing weight is 70% nutrition and 30% exercise. However, it's probably closer to 90% nutrition and 10% exercise. Exercise puts the icing on the cake. It makes you feel amazing. It gets you strong, lean, toned, fit and strong. It improves the health of your bones and heart.

And it increases your metabolism. What you eat (and don't eat) is what's going to see you shed weight. Exercise can be the easy part. Eating well 24/7 (most of the time) can be the challenging part.

It's not just about losing weight or being able to do more push-ups and getting into great shape. It's about how losing weight and getting into great shape makes you feel emotionally, and how those emotions have a flow-on effect to the rest of your life.

On the flip side, it is also about how being overweight and unfit impacts your life and affects you emotionally. It comes down to self-esteem, confidence and pride in yourself.

These are feelings you carry out into the world and which have a ripple effect on the kind of parent and partner you are, and on the kind of person, you are at work and in your social life. It comes down to being your best self. We all know when we are not being the best version of ourselves, and this can get you down and make us feel less worthy.

It's at these times that people make poor food decisions – the result of stress, tiredness, negative emotions, boredom and unhappiness. We may not even realise we are unhappy, and most people I meet actually don't realise how stressed and time-poor they are. We think it's normal.

In a health-coaching consultation, I often ask people to describe their goals. They might say they want to do things like lose weight, increase fitness or get toned.

If I ask why, the response could be something like: "So I can fit into a size ten dress", or "So I can get six-pack abs and go to the beach", or "So I can get a girlfriend".

If I was to probe and ask why one more time, that's when the real introspection begins and the deeper responses come out.

These responses could be: "So I can be happy, feel more confident and feel good about myself". Many people I work with don't even want to set a goal because they have tried in the past and failed.

There are ways to fix that. We just need to have a little win, and then another, and another. Then we have momentum and you become unstoppable.

Calorie Deficit

The number one rule for weight loss is that you must be in a calorie deficit. This means you must consume fewer calories than you burn.

Think of it over the course of a week, not every single day. Some days you might consume about the same amount of calories as you expend, and on some days you might eat more than you burn.

But for the most part, you need to be in a negative energy balance, which is created by increasing calorie output (through moving more), decreasing energy input (through eating less) – or both. It is extremely hard to lose weight when you consume more calories than you are burning.

Most of the time, if you're not losing weight, then you need to eat less. You could exercise more, but that just requires more time and effort.

I often ask people how many calories they consume in a day and how many they burn in a day. Often, they don't know. This is normal. You're not supposed to know off the top of your head, and part of the education process is understanding these numbers.

Not knowing how many calories you consume and how many you burn forms the crux of the problem. There are other factors at play, however, being in a calorie deficit is recognised as the number one principle required for weight loss.

The occasional calorie surplus doesn't hurt either. If you overeat every now and then, don't beat yourself up! There's a school of thought that says a calorie surplus can actually have positive effects on your metabolism and your weight loss goals, because it makes our body increase the amount of energy it has to burn.

Then, when you return to eating normally the increased energy burn still continues. Just don't stay in the surplus for too long.

Eating light is about more than just weight loss. It's a strategy to attain peak health and to be mentally sharp and have high levels of energy and vitality.

Rather than focus on calories, it can be helpful to think in terms of nutrients. Our body craves nutrients and is primed to search for them. We need high-quality vitamins and minerals to function. When we don't provide our body with the key nutrients it requires the whole process goes haywire.

If we don't receive the nutrition we need we are programmed to keep eating. Try eating different things and monitor how you feel in the hours after consuming certain types of foods.

You might think that eating a salad with avocado, olive oil, and a small amount of chicken isn't overly exciting however it's rich in fibre and packed with nutrients which will reduce the likelihood of food cravings later that day and keep you satisfied for longer.

If you eat 2 slices of toast with vegemite and a flat white there's barely any quality nutrition in there which means the chances of wanting to eat again an hour or two later are greatly enhanced.

Blue Zones

On our planet, there are five areas referred to as 'Blue Zones'. These are places where the inhabitants live happily and healthily, until they are well over 100 years old.

One of these Blue Zones is Okinawa, Japan. Okinawans have a saying: "Hara Hachi Bu", which translates to "Eat until you are eight-tenths full". There's a book called Ikigai which outlines the Japanese secrets to a long and healthy life. The book details how overeating results in a long digestive process that accelerates cellular oxidation and starts wearing down our body.

During this process, molecules known as free radicals are created. Free radicals are normal and necessary, however, in high quantities, they can oxidise our cells, engage in unnecessary side reactions, and put our body under oxidative stress.

This process damages the growth, development and survival of cells in the body, and reduces our life span.

The Body's Two Energy Sources

Another important fundamental of fat loss is that our body has two sources of energy:

- consumed carbohydrates
- stored body fat.

- We burn them in that order.

Many people eat more carbohydrates than necessary and are not as active as they should be. As a result, they are always burning carbs and never burning their stored body fat.

FAT LOSS PROCESS

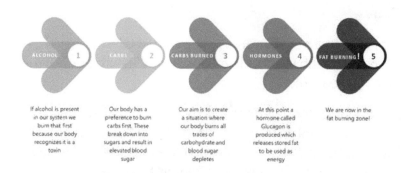

If alcohol is present in our system we burn that first because our body recognizes it is a toxin

Our body has a preference to burn carbs first. These break down into sugars and result in elevated blood sugar

Our aim is to create a situation where our body burns all traces of carbohydrate and blood sugar depletes

At this point a hormone called Glucagon is produced which releases stored fat to be used as energy

We are now in the fat burning zone!

The double-whammy with carbohydrates is that they make us produce the storage hormone insulin, which stores excess carbohydrates as body fat. It takes our body 12 hours to eliminate any carbohydrates we consume, and it is only after this time that we can burn fat.

This is why a lower carbohydrate intake can be beneficial for fat loss. It is also why not eating in the morning allows our body to tip into a fat-burning state.

For example, if our last meal of the day is at 8pm, we cannot burn any fat until 8am the next day. If any carbs are consumed prior to 8am, our body immediately gets to work burning them, and body fat is spared (not burned).

Educational Tips on Health and Weight Loss

Below is a selection of tips and educational snippets regarding health and weight loss. You'll find some of the tips are repeated but in a different way or from a different angle. This is to help you gain a more complete understanding of the given issue.

1. Eat less to create a calorie deficit most of the time

Often, in health and life as a whole, it can be helpful to think in terms of evolution. Human beings are not designed to eat breakfast, morning tea, lunch, afternoon tea, dinner and supper. We are not supposed to eat 24/7. By doing so, it places enormous pressure on our digestive system, one of the most taxing bodily processes.

When we are continually digesting, especially carbohydrates, our blood sugar is constantly elevated, preventing fat-burning and leading to weight gain. It also does not allow time for our immune system to function the way it needs to, because so much energy is tied up in the digestion process. Our body appreciates having a break from constantly digesting food.

This is where a non-eating window of 16 hours can be a smart strategy to implement. My recommendation is that this is done from 8pm until midday the following day, anywhere from two to seven days per week.

Back in the hunter/gatherer days, humans were lucky if they ate a couple of times per day. Even then, we had to catch and prepare our food, which was unprocessed. And as a species, we were a lot more active. Think about the slimmest people in the world and see if you can identify some common traits – they usually eat light and move a lot.

I had a personal training client, Kerry, who was a successful, corporate type. She felt she was eating well, and said she was exercising consistently, three times a week, for 30 minutes each time. I explained to her that this amount of exercise was not enough to compensate for the 50 hours she spent sitting at her desk each week and the 56 hours she spent sleeping – in addition to the calories she was consuming over the course of a week.

To lose weight, Kerry had to increase her energy output or decrease her energy input. Kerry also ended up with an approach to eating where (in her words) she said no, more than she said yes.

We tend to think of our stomachs as petrol tanks – when we eat, we think it needs to be full. It doesn't. Hippocrates said that the best medicine is fasting. Mark Twain said a little starvation can do more for us than the best medicine and the best doctors. If you are hungry, eat something small to quieten the stomach.

Eat light. Eat less.

You will feel better when you do. If you enjoy a flat white, don't have it in addition to your breakfast - make it your breakfast. People still equate food with energy. The irony is that when you eat less, you will have more energy.

2. Get your nutrition right and do what you like for exercise

There is often a debate surrounding the best way to exercise in order to achieve optimal health and your ideal weight. Bearing in mind that nutrition is 90% responsible for results in these areas, once you find and implement the nutrition strategies outlined here, you can do your preferred forms of exercise and not worry about what some people think you should or should not be doing for exercise.

Gyms are full of people who exercise six or seven days per week but don't lose weight because they don't have their nutrition right. Anyone can exercise for 45 minutes a day, and a lot of people enjoy it. Proper nutrition requires education and an element of discipline.

People often smash themselves with exercise and proudly point to their Fitbit and say they burned 400 calories... then go and eat 800 calories at their next meal. An area where people also come undone is snacking. 150 calories here, 200 calories there...and drinking 500 calories per day in the form of coffee, alcohol, juices or soft drinks. It all adds up.

Long, regular bouts of high-intensity exercise actually increase your appetite, making it harder to eat well. Not to mention that exercise of this nature also results in muscle loss, meaning you can lose weight on the scales but actually look less toned and end up weaker, with an increased body fat percentage and a decreased metabolism.

Exercising super hard is rarely enjoyable for the long term. Low-impact exercise and the right nutrition strategy achieves better fat-loss results and is kinder and smarter for your body.

People love different forms of exercise – yoga, walking their dog, weight training, running up and down sand hills, Pilates, swimming. I am passionate about simply being active. All forms of exercise have benefits. When it comes to our body — mobility, strength, flexibility, fitness — it really is a case of 'use it or lose it'. My only criteria for fat loss is that resistance training should be a part of your weekly regimen because of the benefits it has for your metabolism and muscle tone.

Metabolism, in a nutshell, is the rate at which your body burns energy. Our aim is to increase this rate. Boatloads of cardio exercise burns muscle.

The muscle loss actually reduces your metabolism, meaning long, frequent bouts of cardio are not the best long-term weight management solution.

When you want to lose weight, in order of importance, you should look at:

1. nutrition
2. resistance training
3. cardio

You will know your nutrition is working in the best way for you when you are living life at the weight you want, and it's easy. From there, you can feel free to enjoy whatever forms of physical activity you choose to engage in. After all, an exercise program filled with things you dislike is not going to last very long.

I've said this before and I keep repeating it because it is true, yet many people continue not to understand it.

> In most initial consultations with new clients,
> they want to talk about exercise in order
> to get in shape. Then I ask them what their goals are.
> When they say weight loss, we spend the next
> 30 minutes discussing nutrition, because
> what you eat is 90% responsible for what you weigh.
>
> - Scott Capelin

3. The body burns carbs before fat

When it comes to weight loss, aside from the calorie deficit, the fact that the body burns carbs before the fat is one of the biggest, most significant principles of them all. I talked about this earlier in this chapter (*The Body's Two Energy Sources*), and I'm going to revisit the concept again here to flesh it out more.

At the most basic level, our body has two fuel sources: the carbohydrates we consume and the fat on our body. When carbohydrates are present in our system, they are broken down into glucose and float around in the form of blood sugar which is burned first before the body burns body fat.

If it makes it simpler for you, just tell yourself that your body burns the food you eat, before it can burn the stored body fat you carry.

If you regularly consume meals that contain carbohydrates, you will always have an element of blood sugar and always be burning these sugars instead of body fat. In order to burn body fat, we must create an internal environment where our body has the chance to burn off most traces of glucose, so our blood sugar is low.

This can be achieved by reducing the amount of carbohydrates in our diet, and potentially incorporating fasting. When our body runs out of carbs to burn, it switches to its other fuel source – body fat. If you want to lose weight, this must happen – and happen often!

This process is called 'dietary-induced ketosis' and basically means our nutrition strategy results in low blood sugar, so we have to use body fat for energy.

To illustrate this – the body burning body fat over carbohydrates stored as glucose in the blood – I'll share Gail's story. Frustrated with her inability to lose weight, during our initial consultation, Gail explained that she exercised religiously at 6am every morning.

Everything also appeared to be in order with her daily nutrition. I was stumped for a moment and asked if there was any information she had left out. She said, "Before my exercise every morning, I have a protein shake". I asked her what type of shake it was, and we looked it up on the internet. It was a meal replacement shake that contained 70 grams (280 calories) of carbohydrates. I said, "Gail, you don't need a personal trainer, just stop having that shake before your morning exercise session.

The carbs in the shake are elevating your blood sugar and stopping the fat-loss process". Gail stopped having the shake and lost ten kilograms in the following six weeks.

There's a difference between a protein shake and a meal replacement drink. Meal replacements generally have more carbs and more calories, and a protein shake contains protein with no carbs or fat, therefore better for fat loss.

There's also a saying: *When* you eat can be more important than *what* you eat.

Gail's shake had way too many carbs; however, a similar shake would be okay as a mid-afternoon snack, just not first thing in the morning. Loading up on carbs as soon as you get up is the last thing to do if you want to lose weight.

It's okay if you are training for a performance-based event, like a marathon or a triathlon, when weight loss is not the goal. Sometimes, people tell me they wake up and have breakfast cereal with milk and a banana. I tell them that's the breakfast we might prescribe for someone who does not want to lose weight.

I played semi-professional rugby league for a number of years and I would have a breakfast like that to help me gain weight!

It is worthwhile to also note that vegetarians and vegans often find it challenging to reduce the number of carbohydrates they consume in relation to protein and fat.

Their protein options are limited, meaning all they are left with is carbs and vegetarian protein options – which quite often contain carbs. Carbs are not the enemy, it's just that with the way our supermarkets are stocked these days, carbs and sugars are prevalent everywhere.

4. The body burns alcohol before carbs

Here's the real kicker! Our body will burn alcohol before it burns carbs, and then our poor old body fat gets burned last – if at all.

Alcohol is a toxin. Our body recognises this and wants to burn it immediately. Alcohol is high in calories, so it can take a while to burn off. A glass of wine has 200 calories and two glasses are equivalent to a 40-minute run, a spin class, or an hour of hard exercise.

One of the worst things we can do is have two drinks per night because our body has to burn the alcohol, then get to the carbs, and then hopefully get a chance to burn body fat.

I worked with Penelope for seven years. When I first met her, she weighed 74 kilograms and wanted to get to 60 kilograms. For two years, her exercise regimen was flawless.

She exercised frequently, never missed a session, and enjoyed it very much. In addition, her nutrition was perfect – carbohydrates, protein, fat and water intake were all spot on. The problem? Penelope drank a bottle of wine every night.

Due to sheer persistence, and the high quality of her exercise and nutrition, Penelope still managed to lose six kilograms and get down to 68 kilograms.

Then something interesting happened. Her relationship of ten years ended.

As it turned out, her partner was the person she drank with each night. Penelope met a new man who didn't drink, and her bottle-per-night habit ceased.

Within three months, she went from 68 kilograms to 60 kilograms, and has remained there for the past ten years.

This story raises two other points:

- Most people have a weakness somewhere, and it is probably the thing holding them back.
- The people you spend the most time with, have a big impact on your behaviour and results.

5. If you eat too many carbs (and overall calories) and are not active enough, it's a recipe for weight gain

Let's take a look at how weight gain occurs.

As I explained, when we consume carbohydrates, we produce the hormone, insulin. Insulin has a couple of roles and one of them is to help our cells absorb glucose to reduce blood sugar. Long-term high levels of blood sugar affect our body's internal processes and can lead to type 2 diabetes. When this happens, people have to inject themselves with insulin to help the body do what it should do naturally.

Insulin is also a storage hormone. Our body is a very efficient energy-storing machine. Earlier, I said it can be useful to think in terms of evolution. Think about life as it might have been 300,000 years ago. Food was not in abundance. To eat, we had to 'catch' our food, or only eat food that was in season.

We didn't have the luxury of eating regularly. We didn't know where the next meal was coming from or when the next famine would occur. As a result, we evolved to store energy. When we had the chance to feast, our bodies would store the excess energy as fat, which kept us going through lean times.

This genetic survival mechanism doesn't serve us so well with a 24/7 convenience store in every suburb and fast-food stores readily available. In modern society, we are not at the same risk of famine, or of going long periods without food as our prehistoric ancestors did.

Also, the desire to seek sweet, high-calorie foods is in our DNA because it's the most efficient way of sustaining survival.

No wonder it's a challenge to walk out of a supermarket without making impulse purchases.

To summarise:

- Consuming more carbs than we need results in weight gain, and we don't need many carbs
- Food marketing tells us we need carbohydrates for energy, but you will actually have greater energy levels if you eat smaller, lighter meals
- Sugar is a carbohydrate (and also a preservative), and is in most processed foods
- Processed food comes in a packet, or has a barcode, or is still edible after sitting on the shelf for eight months – or all of these

- When we consume carbohydrates they convert to glucose, which is a form of sugar. Our body stores excess glucose as fat
- Think about the food you eat most days. Is it real food, or is it an edible food-like substance?

Many people in Western societies are consuming more calories than they require and are not active enough. This is a recipe for 'weight creep' – where you gain a small amount of weight each year for ten or 20 years, then ask yourself how you became so overweight.

6. Fat loss versus weight loss

Here's a fun fact: The average total weight of all the bones in your skeletal structure is around two kilograms for women and three kilograms for men. Not much, hey! And we can't change this weight. In addition to that, our bone marrow weighs another two to three kilograms, and our body is 60% water.

This is a good time to distinguish between fat loss and weight loss. Weight loss is the more widespread term; however, our goal really should be to lose fat.

Our body is made up of muscles, fat, blood, fluid, bones, teeth and organs. The main ones we can control through exercise and nutrition are muscle and fat. Body composition refers to the ratio of muscle and fat in our body. For example, if someone is 100 kilograms and has a body fat ratio of 30%, put simply, we can say this person has 30 kilograms of fat mass and 70 kilograms of fat-free mass.

A large portion of your fat-free mass is muscle. Muscle is responsible for your metabolism. As mentioned earlier, metabolism can be defined as the rate at which our body burns energy. You have probably heard of having a fast or slow metabolism. The aim is to increase, or at least maintain, your metabolic rate.

Here's an example of what I mean. Carolyn told me she was interested in working with a personal trainer. She said she had recently married, and before her wedding, she didn't eat for eight weeks, did lots of cardio and lost eight kilograms.

She hit her goal weight but felt she looked a little gaunt, and still felt soft and not toned. Shortly after her wedding, Carolyn went on a four-week honeymoon and gained 14 kilograms. The day after she returned from her honeymoon was the day I met her.

What happened with Carolyn's weight loss?

In cases where people lose weight through unhealthy, unsustainable methods, with diet and cardio, or with diet and no resistance training, studies show that the weight lost showing on the scales is 25% fluid, 25% fat and 50% muscle.

In Carolyn's case, this means that before her wedding, she lost two kilograms of water, two kilograms of fat and four kilograms of muscle.

Carolyn's metabolic rate would have been significantly lower after her eight-kilogram, starvation/cardio, weight-loss strategy, because she lost four kilograms of muscle.

Then she took her soft body and sluggish metabolism on a four-week holiday and gained back all the weight she had lost, plus some. After I explained this, she began the process of returning to a healthy weight she was happy with, in a way that was sustainable and would ensure she didn't fluctuate again.

Her program included regular resistance training, low to moderate intensity cardio, and eating a sensible amount of calories with an optimal ratio of carbohydrates, protein and fats.

If someone loses weight via a form of starvation, they'll regain the weight. If they try to do it again, the same way – severe calorie restriction, cardio and no resistance training – it won't have the same weight loss effect as it did the first time, plus there will be further damage to the metabolism and the ability to remain at a healthy, stable body weight, long-term.

A lot of the work I do with people revolves around turning their bodies into a 'metabolic furnace'.

7. Intermittent fasting brings fast results

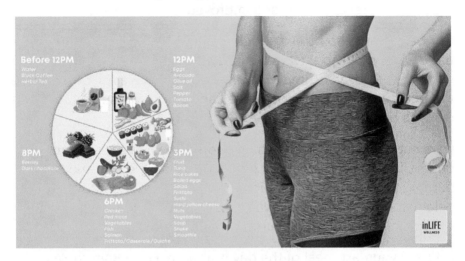

'Intermittent fasting' is not exactly a diet but more of an eating pattern where you cycle between periods of eating and not eating. There are a few different approaches to intermittent fasting:

- a 24-hour fast once or twice a week
- the 16/8 method – eat all meals within eight hours and don't eat for the other 16 hours
- eating for six hours, followed by 18 hours off
- eating all food within four hours and having a 20-hour non-eating window
- the 5:2 method– eat normally for five days and consume only 500 calories on two other non-consecutive days.

According to healthline.com, by reducing your calorie intake, each of these methods should cause weight loss, as long as you don't compensate by overeating during the eating periods. Many people find the 16/8 method to be the simplest, most sustainable and easiest to stick to. It's also the most popular.

As you can see above, there are several ways to do intermittent fasting. All of them split the day or week into eating and fasting periods. The human body did not evolve to eat six meals a day. Instead, we need to give our body regular breaks from the process of digestion to achieve weight loss, greater vitality and improved general health.

Our best chance to burn through the carbs we've eaten during the day is while we sleep. It takes our body up to 12 hours to burn through our carbs, which are stored in our liver and muscles as glycogen. Once the body has burned through the carbs we've consumed, then it's ready to burn body fat.

If we eat a breakfast containing carbohydrates, or eat as soon as we get up, it puts the body back into carb-burning mode and we stop burning fat. This is why skipping breakfast or fasting until midday is helpful for fat loss, because we're providing our bodies with a bigger window of opportunity to burn fat.

Let's say your last meal of the day is at 8pm. From 8pm to 8am, the body is burning up all traces of sugar. From 8am to 12pm, assuming you've not eaten anything, the body is in a massive state of fat burning. Up until midday, you can consume black coffee, black tea, herbal tea and water because these contain no sugars and will not tip your body out of fat-burning mode. All meals you consume should be between 12pm and 8pm.

Some people say, "I couldn't possibly miss breakfast". If this is you, and if you haven't tried intermittent fasting before, just give it a go. It's hard at first, and you'll miss your toast with peanut butter, but it's better than dying early, isn't it? Skip breakfast to accelerate your weight loss results and improve your overall health.

The beauty of intermittent fasting is that it transcends dietary preferences. You could be vegetarian or vegan. You might follow religious protocols, be on a ketogenic diet or enjoy the Paleo diet. You can still incorporate fasting. It is also a calorie reduction strategy in itself because skipping a meal and confining your eating to an eight-hour window, automatically cuts out 30% of your daily calories.

Intermittent fasting is cheap, simple and flexible, as it does not matter which eight-hour window you choose to eat in. Many people also report that after a short time practising intermittent fasting, they become less hungry. It's almost like eating early in the day makes you want a mid-morning snack, then lunch, then afternoon tea, then dinner, and then something after dinner. I am one of four children and my mother has eleven grandchildren. When it comes to babies, she has a saying: "The more they sleep, the more they sleep". I think it's the same with food – the more you eat, the more you eat.

I work with a lovely and successful man in the finance sector called Paul. He'd never had a problem with exercise adherence, but was partial to a beer or wine and had never really grasped the fact that bread, rice and pasta are not overly nutritious. It all affected his ability to lose weight and was thwarting his efforts in the gym. Like most people, Paul always ate an early breakfast - not because he was hungry, but because that's what he had done since he was two years old. I had seen Paul's weight fluctuate over the years but overall, he was robust and healthy.

Paul and I discussed intermittent fasting. At first, he looked at me like I was an alien. Then, he became open to it. Twice a week, he would wait until 10am to have his first meal. Just by doing this, the kilos fell off. Then he extended his fast and didn't start eating until 1:30pm and his two days of fasting each week increased to four. He dropped more weight.

For Paul, what started as an unusual and mildly challenging fasting practice, became easy and enjoyable.

On the mornings Paul doesn't have breakfast, he has two black coffees with a dash of milk and then drinks water. At 53 years old, Paul has gone from 136 kilograms to 101 kilograms and is now the lightest he has been since high school. Sometimes, his first meal at 2pm is a flat white and a Danish. While that isn't loaded with vitamins, minerals and nutrients, his remarkable weight loss results illustrate he has his overall weekly calorie intake under control, and the timing of eating is more important than what is eaten.

Would eggs, avocado and blueberries be a better option? Yes.

Is that going to happen every day? No.

Is losing 35 kilograms of body fat better for your health? Absolutely!

A similar thing happened with Robyn. A successful magazine editor in her 50's, Robyn was going through menopause and showing the early symptoms of Type 2 diabetes.

Fasting saw her go from 113 kilograms to 90 kilograms, which is amazing for someone who spent the previous three decades struggling to lose even a little bit of weight.

That's the power of intermittent fasting just a few times each week. When you try it yourself, you will see the wonders.

8. Get it right 80% of the time

We are all going to 'blow it' or 'slip up' with our nutrition, and probably quite regularly! This is fine – it's called life!

If we apply the Pareto Principle, also known as the 80/20 rule, we can still achieve amazing results – even with slip-ups. The 80/20 rule states that 20% of what we do gets 80% of the results. What health initiatives are covered by the 20%?

- A lower-carb diet, offset by increasing our consumption of natural fats and protein
- Fasting until midday a few times per week, and especially after a night out, a big dinner or a big weekend of food
- Exercising regularly, including some form of resistance training every week
- 10,000+ steps per day

Your nutrition strategy should be sustainable, enjoyable, results-oriented and effortless. It should not be a chore. It should be a lifestyle.

When I talk to my successful health coaching clients, I often ask them what they believe are the 20% of things they do that get 80% of their results.

More often than not they say eating all meals between 12pm and 8pm and exercising four or five times per week. It really can be as simple as that.

9. A higher-fat, lower-carb diet leads to fat loss

Eating a high-fat, low-carb diet is one of the most important, yet least understood, counterintuitive concepts in weight loss.

When we consume fat, it suppresses the production of insulin. (Remember how we said insulin is a storage hormone that results in a fat gain?) If we inhibit our ability to store fat, we are much less likely to gain weight.

That's it! Simple.

So, consuming some fat helps us burn fat by lowering blood sugar, meaning it is less likely to be stored as body fat. When our blood sugar is low, our body switches to its alternative fuel source. It derives its energy from the body fat stored on our arms, thighs, stomach and butt.

Furthermore, the consumption of fat results in the production of a hormone called leptin. Leptin signals to our brain that we are full, so incorporating some fats at each meal makes us feel satisfied and drastically reduces hunger cravings because of the leptin that gets released in our system.

Personally, I know whenever I want to eat something sweet or carb-rich in the afternoon or evening, I can look back and identify a lack of good fat consumption earlier in the day.

A ketogenic diet is one in which up to 80% of daily calories come from fats. This leaves very little room for protein and carbohydrates.

The reason a keto-based approach results in fat loss is because when there are no carbs and sugar in our system, our body has no choice but to burn body fat.

Proponents of the calorie-in/calorie-out approach argue with this, claiming you cannot consume 3,000 calories of fat per day and expect to lose weight. However, a ketogenic diet is renowned for good short-term weight-loss results. It's also renowned for being hard to stick to long term.

We don't have to go to the extremes of getting 80% of our calories from fats as prescribed by the ketogenic approach, but the point is that a ketogenic diet is one that harnesses the effects of forcing the body to derive its energy from body fat because of a lack of carbs; thus, a person loses body fat when they eat according to the ketogenic diet's strict protocols.

It is not that carbs are terrible, it is just that sugar is so prevalent these days, the more low-carb choices we make, the better.

Natural Society is a health research organisation that conducted research into the average consumption of sugar from 1700 to the present day. It found that:

- In 1700, the average person consumed approximately 4.9 grams of sugar each day (1.81 kilograms per year).
- In 1800, the average person consumed approximately 22.4 grams of sugar each day (10.2 kilograms per year).
- In 1900, the average person consumed approximately 112 grams of sugar each day (40.8 kilograms per year).
- In 2009, 50% of Americans consumed approximately 227 grams of sugar each day (81.6 kilograms per year).

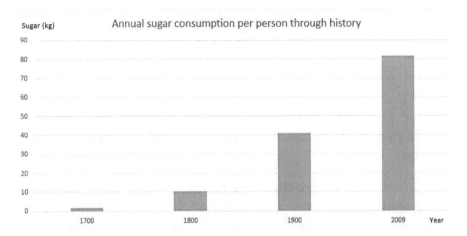

Annual sugar consumption per person through history

10. A higher-fat, lower-carb diet increases mental acuity and energy

Evolution again. It's 400 BCE. You've woken up. You're hungry. No food is in sight, so you go in search. You need to be stealthy and alert to remain safe. Our body has evolved to increase mental sharpness when our carb stores are low.

Modern-day bread and breakfast cereals are mass-produced and high in sugar. Consuming these foods early in the day leads to mid-morning brain fog and the inability to operate at peak mental capacity. Furthermore, sugar is addictive, and breakfast options that are low in nutrients and temporarily satisfying then lead us on the search for more food. Food companies know this and intentionally make foods low in nutrients and unsatisfying for our bodies so we eat more.

Many of my health coaching clients keep a food diary. At the bottom of each page, there is a section to report on areas such as sleep, mood, exercise undertaken and water intake each day. People notice that on the days their sugar intake is high, their mood is low and so is their energy. Generally, many people think carbohydrates give us energy when the opposite is true. By lowering your carbohydrate intake, you will actually have more energy and feel a lot clearer and sharper mentally.

Burning carbs is like burning petrol. We get a quick hit of energy which rapidly dies off. Burning body fat is like burning coal. It's a much more efficient fuel source to operate on and when we do, we feel a lot better.

11. A high-fat diet stabilises blood sugar and cuts out peaks and troughs

Eating foods high in carbohydrates rapidly elevates our blood sugar. After a couple of hours, our blood sugar plummets sharply, and our energy levels rise and fall in line with these blood sugar peaks and troughs. When we reduce the amount of sugar in our diet, these energy fluctuations reduce. We do not want our blood sugar spiking and dropping all day, every day.

The interesting thing about consuming fat-based foods, such as eggs, olive oil, coconut oil, avocado, butter and nuts, is the fats actually suppress the blood sugar spikes, resulting in much smoother energy levels. It is during the sugar slumps that we often crave bad foods and make poor food choices. Increasing the number of natural fats in our diet reduces the likelihood of slumps.

12. Understand the hunger scale

The hunger scale can take some of the confusion out of nutrition. Imagine a line going from left to right, and numbered one to ten. One means you are so hungry, you could chew your arm off. Ten means you are so full you want to fall asleep, a bit like the feeling you have after lunch on Christmas Day. What would be a good word to describe the number five here? People often say 'content' or 'satisfied', which is correct.

On this scale, what is the best number to start eating at? The answer is three. What's the danger of waiting until you get to one before you start eating? You will eat everything in sight!

What number should you stop eating at?

Some people say six, seven, eight or even ten. Some people also say five, which is the correct answer. Think about it. Why would you eat beyond feeling satisfied?

There's probably a reason: maybe because eating brings us pleasure, or maybe because, when you were seven years old, you were told you couldn't leave the table or have your dessert until your plate was empty.

The problem is – you're 48 years old now, and 12 kilograms heavier than you want to be and you're still doing the same thing.

I have a friend called Luke who recently lost five kilograms.

Knowing what I know about nutrition, I commented that he must be eating well. "Not really", he said. "I'm just following the hunger scale."

He said the previous night, he ate two slices of pizza instead of eight.

Using the hunger scale resulted in Luke being in a calorie deficit and allowed his body to burn body fat rather than go into a calorie surplus and contribute to his body fat stores.

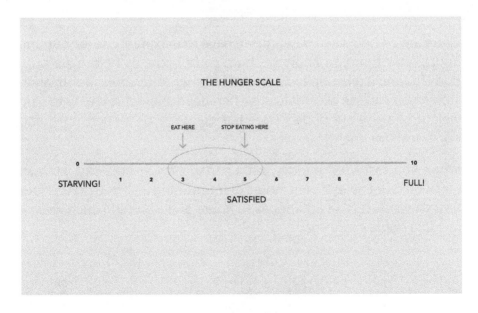

13. Maximise your fat-burning hours

Maximising your fat-burning hours is related to intermittent fasting, which was discussed in point 7 above. It has been mentioned a few times and is worth repeating: our body will burn carbs before body fat, so if we are constantly consuming carbohydrates, we will never burn body fat. Therefore, we need to facilitate a situation where we can 'chew' into our fat stores.

Fasting is a great way to do this. An alternative is to reduce our carbs as already mentioned. If you feel fasting until midday is not for you, try a carb-free breakfast. If you are into fasting, a carb-free breakfast is also great on the days you choose to eat earlier in the day.

An example of a carb-free breakfast is to have eggs — scrambled, fried, poached, boiled or an omelette — with avocado, halloumi, or bacon cooked in olive oil and natural butter. No toast! In a breakfast like this, there are no carbs for our body to burn.

The fat from the egg yolk, avocado, coconut oil and butter further suppresses insulin and lowers blood sugar. This makes our body produce a hormone called glucagon, which enables body fat to be unlocked and released from our fat stores and sent to our bloodstream and muscles to be burned for energy.

There are 24 hours in a day, and we have to maximise the fat-burning hours. Now that you know we burn carbohydrates before we burn body fat, and it takes up to 12 hours to burn through our carbohydrate stores, you can see why fat loss is often not achieved. It is easy to gain weight because our bodies store the excess carbs we consume (and don't need for energy) as fat.

When you fast until midday, rather than having breakfast at 7am, you would get an extra five hours of fat-burning in. If you do this four times a week, it is an additional 20 hours of fat-burning each week – or 1,000 hours every year!

14. Manage expectations for long-term sustainability

In terms of managing expectations and setting ourselves up for success in terms of weight loss and sustaining healthy eating in the long term, it's important to understand:

- there **will** be temptations
- you **will** get hungry
- you **will** eat some rubbish
- you **will** have social occasions where you don't **have** to eat and drink but you might **want** to – and that's fine
- you **will** be unprepared at times and have to do your best with what's available.

Sometimes, you are good for a while, and sometimes you slacken off. It goes in phases. Don't fight it too much. If you're in a bad patch with food, try and work out of it or compensate with the intermittent fasting strategy. Be kind to yourself. We don't want to develop a bad relationship or negative associations with food.

Note: if you have been eating unhealthily for ten years, it's not a phase and it's time to do something about it.

If you feel you've stuffed up, start again. Take a positive step immediately. You may have a huge lunch and then a snack for afternoon tea. Fine – but don't have dinner and have your next meal at midday the following day. Let your body deal with the food you have already consumed. The worst thing to do is eat meals on top of meals, and heap food on top of undigested food that the body is yet to fully process.

15. Who said breakfast is the most important meal of the day?

There is a quote attributed to John Kellogg in 1891, which says, "In many ways, breakfast is the most important meal of the day". He said this when Corn Flakes were first invented. Breakfast is actually the least important meal of the day.

16. Who created the food pyramid?

Large food companies — in particular, those that manufacture and sell bread, rice, pasta and cereals — and massive supermarkets created the food pyramid to make carbohydrates the foundation of our nutrition regimen – because that's what they sell. The original food pyramid, developed in 1980, helped them sell their products. It didn't help us achieve peak health.

I finished high school in 1993 and went to university from 1994 to 1997 to complete a business degree. My first corporate role was with one of Australia's largest supermarket chains. I was in the Marketing and Management Department, so I saw food marketing at its most conniving.

The food pyramid may have contributed to the overweight epidemic we have today. To our credit, at least we have done what we were told – we just didn't realise, at the time, we were told the wrong thing.

Have a think about the types of foods in the pyramid below. It recommends that two-thirds of your diet be comprised of carbohydrates, yet the foundation of it all is processed foods devoid of nutrition.

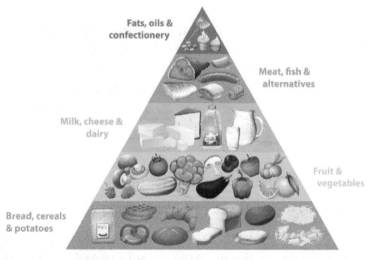

In recent years, there has been a shift towards replacing the food pyramid with MyPlate.

The image below illustrates this revised approach. It is still flawed because it recommends three-quarters of our calories come from carbohydrates and there is no mention of nutritious natural fats.

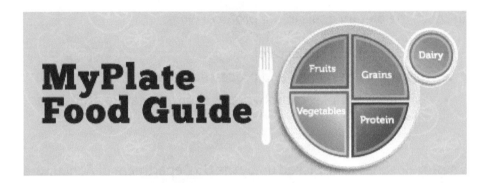

17. How did the low-fat movement originate?

In 1958, an American scientist called Ancel Keys devised a research program called 'The Seven Countries Study'. It examined the association between diet and cardiovascular disease in different countries. The study revealed that the countries where fat consumption was the highest had the most heart disease, supporting the idea that dietary fat causes heart disease.

The problem lies in what was left out, including:

- countries where people eat a lot of fat but have little heart disease, such as Holland and Norway
- countries where fat consumption is low, but the rate of heart disease is high, such as Chile.

Basically, only data from countries that supported the theory was used – a process known as cherry-picking. This observational study gained massive media attention and had a major influence on dietary guidelines for the next few decades.

In 1977, an American committee of the US Senate, led by George McGovern, published the first *Dietary Goals for the United States* to reverse the country's heart disease epidemic. These guidelines received major criticism at the time from the American Medical Association and many respected scientists, like John Yudkin, who insisted that sugar was to blame for rising heart disease in the USA.

In short, the dietary goals in the protocol were:

- eat less fat and cholesterol
- consume less refined and processed sugars
- eat more complex carbohydrates from vegetables, fruits and grains.

These guidelines were picked up by the US Department of Agriculture (USDA) and resulted in a low-fat, high-carb diet for everyone. The guidelines were based on observational studies and had no scientific proof to back them up, despite being conducted by scientists.

Since then, many randomised, controlled trials have shown this dietary approach doesn't really work for the people it was meant to help. An interesting fact is that the obesity epidemic started around the time these guidelines were published and the type 2 diabetes epidemic followed soon after.

18. Common food myths

Here are three common food myths that persist today.

- **Eggs are bad**

For the last 40 years, the same people who brought us the low-fat movement have had us thinking eggs are bad for us because they increase cholesterol. Eggs are actually a superfood – you couldn't get a better combination of protein and natural fat. As with a lot of food these days, choose the eggs you eat carefully – free-range, organic eggs are best.

- **All fat is evil**

As mentioned above, the low-fat movement was created from misinformation that led people to believe fatty foods created heart disease, which isn't entirely true.

Don't you think it's interesting that low-fat foods have been around for 50 years and the Western world is fatter than it has ever been?

You may have heard of the distinction between 'good fats' and 'bad fats'. I prefer to look at it as 'natural fats' and 'man-made fats'.

Natural fats, as the name suggests, are fats that are found naturally and include the visible fat on meat, nuts, avocado and olive oil. These are great to eat.

Man-made fats are the saturated fats and trans-fat found in chocolate, margarine and fast food – best avoided.

- **Drink milk for calcium**

Milk is great if you are a baby cow trying to gain 600 kilograms in 18 months, and drinking it from your mother's udder. The milk in containers at our local supermarket has very little resemblance to the milk that comes from cows. It is also a little strange that, as adults, we are drinking milk beyond weaning, and that it is the milk from another mammal.

One of the most fundamental recommendations for weight loss is to reduce or eliminate dairy. Milk contains a type of protein called casein which is difficult for our body to deal with.

The digestive process is affected and weight gain (or preventing weight loss) can be the end result.

19. Burning carbs is like burning petrol, and burning fat is like burning coal

There are times during the day when we may feel we are in a slump. We have been led to believe we need some carbs as a pick-me-up. This isn't the greatest solution as it was probably the consumption of sugary carbs that put you in the slump.

As previously mentioned, burning carbs is like burning petrol – it makes us feel good temporarily; however, very soon we are back where we started and looking for another energy boost.

Burning fat is like burning coal. When we allow our body to become a fat-burning machine, rather than a sugar-burning machine, we are better-fueled for longer and we have more energy, fewer food cravings and we think more clearly.

20. Food has changed over the last 100 years

In terms of genetic evolution, the human body has hardly changed at all over the last 300,000 years. But the food we now eat would be quite unrecognisable to our ancestors. Walk into any supermarket and it is bursting with processed foods and edible, food-like substances, containing sugar and preservatives, that our body does not recognise as food.

It is not surprising that after a lifetime of eating such foods, horrific diseases manifest. One in two men will get cancer, and one in three women. This is not normal!

The solution here is simple in theory, but harder to implement. Eat natural, unprocessed foods — organic or locally sourced if possible. Eggs, fruit, vegetables, meat, nuts … you can see why the Paleo diet is so popular.

21. A useful hormone summary

Work with your hormones to burn fat.

- Insulin: Produced by the pancreas and released when carbohydrates are consumed. Designed to reduce blood sugar and also store excess carbohydrates as fat

- Glucagon: Also produced in the pancreas and released into the bloodstream when our blood sugar is low. Glucagon releases our stored body fat to be used for energy. This is a good thing!

- Ghrelin: This hormone is produced in our stomach and lets us know we are hungry, encouraging us to eat. When we eat foods that are not nutritious, we are prompted to eat more

- Leptin: It is actually produced in our fat cells and signals to the brain that we are full. Our goal is to produce this often, so we remain satisfied for longer and, therefore, eat less and reduce cravings

22. Figure it out for yourself!

The most powerful way to take control of your health long term is to figure out what works for you. I have seen thousands of people achieve mind-blowing transformations in terms of weight loss and improving their overall health, and I may have offered them support, accountability and guidance, however, I can honestly say that I did not write diet plans for them all.

Regardless of how long someone works with a coach, they probably won't work with them forever, which is why knowing and understanding the right approach for you is critical to staying in shape for the next few decades.

Dieters almost always fail because they have this very wrong belief that there is a perfect diet out there somewhere that they just need to find. The truth? No matter what Keto Kyle, Paleo Pauley, Fasting Fred or Vegan Vera try to tell you, there is no such thing as the perfect diet.

Those who are successful don't discover a diet; rather, they create the right diet for themselves. They don't follow a diet; they build a lifestyle that fits their unique physiology, psychology, and personal preferences so that it's sustainable for life.

They do this by using a methodology and mind-set very different from what's typical. Rather than focusing on what's currently in vogue, they focus on their own body's reaction. They don't study books, blogs, podcasts, food lists and research, they study themselves.

They do it through trial and error and slowly build a lifestyle while simultaneously giving up short-term dieting.

We humans are funny; we realize in most other worthwhile endeavors that mastery is a process, not a recipe. In other words, if you want to be a great pianist, there is no procedure you follow from start to finish that provides a linear and predictable outcome. The process is individual and has ups and downs, peaks and valleys, with great triumphs followed by frustrating failures. All along the way we learn, practice, and master the steps until we become proficient. This process of practicing to achieve mastery is an individual journey we all must make, and it applies to health & fitness too. If you really want to change, you will give up being the dieter and become a metabolic detective instead.

- Jade Teta

Spend time educating yourself and experimenting with different approaches and after a while the results become effortless.

What Type of Exercise Should I Do?

In this book, I talk a lot about being in great physical shape as that is my first and foremost approach to health. There are hundreds of other things we can do for our health, which are all valid, that I have not touched on here.

There's massage, having a colonic, meditation, acupuncture, seeing a naturopath, chiro, physio, osteopathy, gut health, detox, infra-red sauna … the list goes on.

A broader question might be: What does wellness (or well-being) mean to you? Well-being could touch on the emotional, mental, physical and spiritual elements of living your best life.

Overall wellness includes all these elements: your social life, financial position, the level of autonomy and creativity in your life, your spiritual beliefs, stress levels, travel, adventure, fun, optimism, contributing to society, having a positive attitude, maintaining a fulfilling relationship, doing work that inspires you, living in a home you love, feeling important, self-confidence, life balance, personal development, looking and feeling great and having strong connections with friends and family.

For the most part, however, this book focuses on physical well-being.

Being in shape resolves a whole host of health considerations. It involves regular exercise or a high level of activity, and a healthy diet. This makes you look good, feel great and have loads of energy. It also increases bone density and reduces the risk of heart disease, cancer and weight-related illnesses.

And being in shape makes you feel comfortable within yourself, which results in a plethora of positive emotions such as increased self-esteem, improved self-image, pride, happiness, increased mental strength, resilience and fortitude. Exercising is a physical and mental outlet, and very often, it's the only time you get each day to do something for yourself.

These days, most health issues relate to heart health and weight-related illnesses, which is why the foundation of peak health is being in great physical shape. Through my work, I see people become lighter, stronger, and more flexible, with increased physical stamina and endurance.

I am yet to see a person in peak physical shape who does not feel incredible. This leads to the question: *What type of exercise should I do?*

You may be thinking this is going to be a lengthy section, and it could be. However, I am keeping it brief.

The best long-term exercise regimens are the ones you enjoy. It doesn't matter how good something is for you because if you don't enjoy your weekly exercise plan, there's a good chance it will not last long.

If your goal is to live at a healthy weight, remember that nutrition is 90% of this. Exercise is just the icing on the cake. If you get your nutrition right, you can do what you like for exercise.

Eating in the manner outlined throughout this book can help get you to a healthy weight. However, it does not make you fit, strong, or flexible. Exercise does that.

Your entire health and wellness picture can not be completed by just one mode or method of exercise. If all you do is walk every day, you will lack strength. If you only lift heavy weights, you won't work the smaller muscles and will run the risk of injury, and you won't be aerobically fit .

If you only do yoga, you won't stimulate your metabolism as much as you could by incorporating more resistance training. If you only do Pilates, you will get strong in a certain way, such as having a strong core and strengthening smaller muscles but lack strength in other areas.

And if you have no balance or mobility, it doesn't matter how fit or strong you are, you will blow over in a stiff wind, or fall over if you trip on something.

Many people have been conditioned to believe you have to smash yourself with high-intensity exercise to achieve good results.

You do not!

There are much smarter, more enjoyable and sustainable ways to exercise. In fact, the higher the intensity of the cardiovascular exercise you do, the more muscle you burn.

This lowers your metabolism, reduces strength, and reduces muscle tone. Exercising frequently at a high intensity can produce more cortisol (the stress hormone), and your appetite will increase from the harder training. Altogether, it's not a good combination!

The Ideal Exercise Combination

I spent years training fitness models – they don't do ten-kilometre road runs. Instead, they do the right kind of resistance training, their nutrition is spot on and they do low-intensity cardio. It is the perfect recipe for fat loss and achieving the body shape you're after.

Plus, it allows you to remain injury-free, and it's enjoyable and sustainable. Nobody wants to wake up each day dreading their upcoming workout because you know it's going to be exhausting.

I meet a lot of people in their 30's, 40's, 50's and 60's who have done years of high-intensity exercise and are now looking for a more sustainable, low-impact, enjoyable and body-friendly exercise regimen.

It's a bit of a mental shift to do exercise that does not involve heavy weights or getting your heart rate so high that you are close to vomiting, and clients are often surprised when the results are better.

I see so many people exercising ten times a week. Not only do their bodies not change physically, but they sometimes become worse. This is a result of the types of training they do and the way they eat. I also see people who exercise three or four times a week and have their nutrition spot on.

They manage to keep their bodies in good condition for the long term.

To be in great shape, the three variables, in order of importance, are:

1. nutrition
2. resistance training
3. cardio

We've discussed nutrition already in previous chapters, so will move on to the other two — resistance training and cardio.

Resistance Training

One important recommendation for your weekly exercise regime is some form of resistance training. Resistance training is a broad term that involves placing your muscles under some kind of positive stress. The technical definition is: to expose the muscular-skeletal system to loads greater than those experienced in daily life.

We can use our body weight for resistance, or we can use weights, machines or bands. Yoga and Pilates are also forms of resistance training. Weight training is a type of resistance training.

Resistance training is like the fountain of youth. Undergoing a resistance training session stimulates hormones, such as testosterone and growth hormones, produces collagen, makes you burn more fat which results in a lean, toned appearance, and releases endorphins, which are positivity hormones.

Resistance training prevents muscle loss and stimulates your metabolism. Remember, one definition of metabolism is 'the rate at which your body burns energy', so it stands to reason that if we want to lose body fat, an increased metabolism is a good thing.

This is why anyone who wants to lose weight should be doing some form of resistance training.

In my first consultation with Danielle, she mentioned that six months ago, she went on a three-week juice fast and lost six kilograms. I didn't respond. After a ten-second pause, she said, "In the following month, I gained seven kilograms".

What happened to Danielle is her metabolism slowed down due to the muscle and fluid she lost when she dropped the six kilograms on the juice fast. Next, when she went off the juice fast (essentially a starvation diet) and ate normally again, she regained the weight with a little extra. After you've slowed your metabolism in this way, it is harder to lose the regained weight because your metabolic rate is still low.

When we eat for weight loss or to maintain a healthy weight, we need to couple this with regular weekly resistance training to avoid losing muscle. If you lose muscle, you can lose weight on the scales and still not appear any more toned, and of course, you lose strength.

The goal is to lose body fat while maintaining muscle levels. This way, you will look better, feel better, be stronger, and set yourself up for long-term success by maintaining, or even increasing, your metabolism. This is why you should lift weights if you want to lose weight.

Incorporating resistance training in your exercise plan while you are on a fat-loss diet is the key to preventing muscle loss. You aren't trying to gain boatloads of muscle — we just don't want to lose any either. I see many clients who say they want to lose ten kilograms.

After a few months, they have lost six kilograms, but they look and feel better than ever because they worked on their strength, maintained their muscle mass and improved their body shape. They became lighter, fitter and stronger, and they had more energy!

Body fat takes up three times more space than muscle, so if you can lose body fat and maintain or even gain a bit of muscle, you will significantly improve your body shape and lose centimetres from your waist and hips — even if the number on the scales doesn't seem to reduce drastically.

Most people have tried to lose weight at some point in the past, and more often than not, it probably involved some kind of dieting and calorie restriction, combined with cardio. This method usually results in weight loss, meaning the number on the scales goes down. But you need to consider the big question: What kind of weight was lost?

Our bodies can lose three things: fluid, body fat and muscle. If our goal is to lose body fat, along with that, there will be some fluid loss, which is generally associated with a decrease in water retention and bloating. This happens when sugar intake is decreased, because excess carbohydrate consumption can result in fluid retention.

Many people who lose weight actually lose up to 50% muscle. This is bad in the medium and long term when they go off the diet or reduce their exercise.

Why?

Because, at this point, the weight creeps back up to the original weight, plus some more, and then it is harder to lose because of the way the metabolism has been negatively affected as a result of the way the weight was lost in the first place.

Again, this is why resistance training is a key component of a fat-loss diet. (Note the term fat-loss as opposed to weight-loss.) Resistance training combined with eating less and moving more is the best long-term weight management strategy.

Most people are focused on the number of calories they burn during an exercise session. In a challenging workout, you might burn around 300 calories.

The massive benefit of a resistance training session is the way your metabolism remains elevated for the 36 hours after the session is completed, resulting in a higher than normal calorie burn during that period, compared to not doing a resistance training session.

Considering your muscle mass is responsible for your metabolism, if you can gain some muscle, you will also burn more fat 24/7 and be able to get away with a more relaxed diet.

If you are a woman, please do not worry about bulking up. It is hard for a man to gain muscle, but it's much harder for a woman because females don't have as much testosterone as males (and testosterone is a key ingredient for building muscle).

In addition, 'muscle gain' and 'fat loss' are two completely different goals, requiring totally opposite nutrition strategies. If you are a woman eating in a calorie deficit, it makes it even harder to gain muscle. So don't worry about looking like a bouncer at a nightclub! It's not likely to happen.

It's important to also note that some body types gain muscle easier than others, and people with these body types can lift lighter weights less regularly for the same outcome.

Muscle gain requires a calorie surplus, so if you feel you are gaining more muscle than you want to, perhaps your calorie intake is too high, or you have the middle body type, the one that gains muscle easiest, in the image below.

THE
BODY TYPES

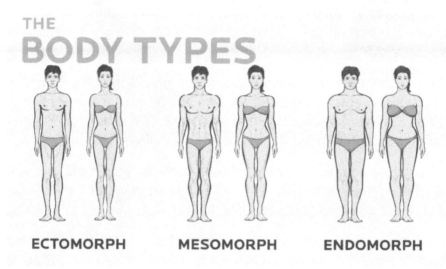

ECTOMORPH   **MESOMORPH**   **ENDOMORPH**

What we are really aiming to achieve while we lose body fat is muscle maintenance. What we don't want is to lose weight where half the loss is muscle.

Most people I meet have a goal to lose a certain amount of weight. After six to 12 months, they may have not lost the amount on the scales they initially set out to lose.

This is because they have lost fat and gained muscle. However, because they lost fat and gained muscle, it doesn't matter that their weight isn't as low as they'd hoped, because they've ended up being in the best shape of their lives, looking and feeling better than ever.

However, some people are the other way — they set out to lose six kilograms, and end up losing ten kilograms pretty easily.

The majority of people I work with say they want to be 'toned'. This means losing fat and maintaining muscle. If you lose muscle as part of the weight loss process, the scales will say you're lighter, but you won't be any more toned.

You can actually be lighter but less toned or lighter with a higher body fat percentage if you lose the wrong kind of weight.

The big takeaway I hope you have gained from the discussion thus far is: to get healthy and stay healthy in the long term, you want to lose body fat and not muscle. Resistance training is essential in helping you do this.

Forms of resistance training include:

- free weights at home or in the gym
- weight training machines (the ones you load up with a pin or weight plates)
- Reformer Pilates
- group exercise classes that involve weights
- yoga
- mat Pilates
- body-weight workouts.

Cardio

In addition to nailing our nutrition and doing some form of resistance training a few times each week, you should aim to be as active as possible! This is where the third part — cardio — comes in.

Cardio exercise can be walking, yoga, swimming, running on the sand, golf, tennis, hiking, horse riding, or doing an indoor cycling class. It's anything that increases your heart rate. Having a job that involves sitting down for 40 to 50 hours per week can put you at a disadvantage.

However, it can be offset by eating less and moving more. Doing 10,000 steps per day pretty much solves many of our health-related problems.

One of the goals of wellness is to live with massive levels of energy and vitality, and a vibrant, positive attitude. The irony of wanting to have more energy is that you have to use more energy!

Another irony is that you have more energy when you eat less — not when you eat more. The body really is a case of 'use it or lose it' when it comes to strength, tone, flexibility, bones, joints and ligaments.

Some people ask if there is an issue with overtraining. I'm not advising you to shoot for the Olympics or train four hours a day — but I am a big fan of training frequently at a moderate intensity.

Train daily, sometimes twice — it's way better than the alternative of not being active enough — and do exercise you enjoy and that helps get the outcomes you want.

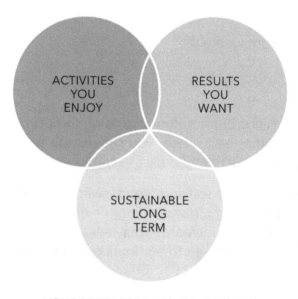

YOUR BEST APPROACH TO EXERCISE

Fasting — The Ultimate Weight Loss and Health Improvement Hack

We touched on fasting in a previous chapter, and because it provides the foundation of what I believe is the most effective approach for weight loss and general health, we are going to double down on it here.

I have been helping people improve their health and fitness for over 20 years. In at least 95% of cases, my clients have a goal of weight loss. It could be a goal of losing three kilograms or 30 kilograms.

Each goal is equally as compelling to the individual, and whether it's three or 30 kilograms, both require the same strategy in terms of exercise and nutrition.

I have owned several health clubs and have done thousands of consultations with new members. It is important to commence with a consultation to get a feel for the client's exercise history, injuries and medical considerations.

A consultation also provides the opportunity to understand the client's lifestyle. We can then discuss and set goals, take measurements and talk about nutrition.

The funny thing is, people often decide to join a gym or see a personal trainer to exercise, but inevitably, when we discuss goals, weight loss is one of them. We'll end up talking a lot about nutrition because that's what is responsible for weight loss — more so than exercise.

You can exercise ten times a week, but if your nutrition isn't right, you'll get fit and strong but you won't lose any weight.

Nutrition is a broad topic that is fascinating, frustrating and intensely personal. I was never a huge proponent of intermittent fasting until around 2014 when — after helping people with weight loss for 15 years — it became very clear that the main issue was overeating. In other words, consuming too many calories over the course of a day, a week or a month.

What I have discovered is eating results in more eating. When someone has a meal before 9 am, they are more likely to eat something else around 11 am, followed by lunch in the middle of the day. it's almost as though eating early in the day breaks the seal and opens the floodgates. Before you know it, they have consumed at least 1,000 calories and only half the day is done.

These days, most foods in supermarkets are low in nutrients and because our body isn't satisfied by low-nutrient foods, we don't even question why we are compelled to eat again a couple of hours after our last meal.

And then we eat again, and then we eat dinner, and then, two hours after dinner, it's not unusual to find ourselves staring into an open fridge or pantry, looking for something to snack on while we relax or because we're bored.

Some people can lose weight by eating anywhere between 1,500 and 2,500 calories per day. Some people need to hit a lower daily calorie intake in order to achieve any kind of significant weight loss.

Determining factors can be your daily activities, exercise frequency, genetics, and level of muscle. As mentioned previously, weight loss generally requires a calorie deficit, or reducing food consumption.

Eating five or six times a day, like the above scenario, makes this challenging. It is not possible to lose weight when you are consistently consuming more calories than you are burning.

Our aim is to burn our stored body fat and use it for energy, and it's almost impossible to do this when our body is constantly burning the food we keep pumping in.

Intermittent fasting — most commonly achieved by eating all your meals between 12pm and 8pm, or any eight-hour window for eating and a 16-hour window of fasting — solves so many issues and can work with whatever nutrition preference you choose.

Fasting is key to increased levels of vitality and energy. You'll feel less bloated, and burn fat rather than sugar.

The benefits of intermittent fasting include:

- **Weight Loss and Fat Burning**

You simply can't eat as many calories in eight hours as you can in 14 hours. In addition, we can only burn fat when carbohydrates are not present.

It takes 12 hours for our bodies to remove all traces of carbs from the blood. So if our last meal of the day is at 8pm, we cannot burn fat until 8am the next day. Between 8 am and midday, when the fast is still going, we have our fat-burning window.

- **Anti-aging**

Digestion is a process that takes up a huge amount of energy. When we let it switch off, a host of other immune functions kick in, resulting in increased production of growth hormone, testosterone and collagen, the way they did in our younger years.

Fasting also lowers insulin levels, therefore reducing the risk of insulin resistance and developing type 2 diabetes. 'Human growth hormone' is an important hormone produced by your pituitary gland and plays a key role in body composition (your levels of muscle and body fat), cell repair and metabolism.

Short-term fasting actually increases your metabolism by anywhere from 3% to 14%, meaning you burn more calories with no additional effort. Growth hormone also boosts muscle growth, strength and exercise performance, while helping you recover from injury and disease.

Low levels of growth hormone may decrease your quality of life, increase your risk of disease and result in weight gain.

Healthline reports that optimal levels are especially important for weight loss, recovery and regular exercise. Fasting is not just a calorie reduction strategy. It assists in weight loss, health and longevity by positively altering our internal environment.

You don't need food for energy. Eating a meal isn't going to give you an abundance of energy.

In fact, the opposite is true. Fasting increases energy. Eat light. Give the body a rest. Allow it to regenerate and slow the aging process.

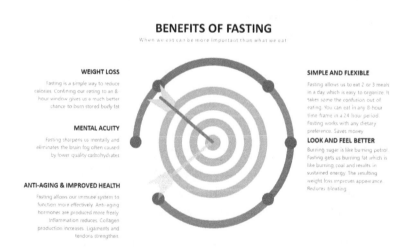

BENEFITS OF FASTING

When we eat can be more important than what we eat

WEIGHT LOSS

Fasting is a simple way to reduce calories. Confining our eating to an 8-hour window gives us a much better chance to burn stored body fat

MENTAL ACUITY

Fasting sharpens us mentally and eliminates the brain fog often caused by lower quality carbohydrates

ANTI-AGING & IMPROVED HEALTH

Fasting allows our immune system to function more effectively. Anti-aging hormones are produced more freely. Inflammation reduces. Collagen production increases. Ligaments and tendons strengthen

SIMPLE AND FLEXIBLE

Fasting allows us to eat 2 or 3 meals in a day which is easy to organize. It takes some the confusion out of eating. You can eat in any 8-hour time frame in a 24 hour period. Fasting works with any dietary preference. Saves money

LOOK AND FEEL BETTER

Burning sugar is like burning petrol. Fasting gets us burning fat which is like burning coal and results in sustained energy. The resulting weight loss improves appearance. Reduces bloating

- **Mental Acuity**

We feel more alert when we don't eat in the morning and don't get the 'brain fog' often associated with early morning carbohydrate consumption. Think in terms of evolution: if we were living 300,000 years ago, and it was 11 am, and we hadn't eaten yet, our mind would need to be at its sharpest to hunt and kill something to eat. The point I'm attempting to make is that our bodies evolved to operate efficiently when we don't eat a carbohydrate-heavy breakfast.

- **Simple and Flexible**

It really is very straightforward — you eat your first meal at midday, a snack in the afternoon if you need it, and dinner at 7 pm. You can even snack after dinner if you can make the 8 pm cut-off.

You don't need to fast until midday every day to achieve weight loss with intermittent fasting, but the more often you do, the better the results.

And, if that timing doesn't fit in with your lifestyle, remember that the eating window does not have to be between 12pm and 8pm, it can be any eight-hour window within a 24-hour period, for example, your eating window could be between 8am and 4pm, and your fasting window from 4pm to 8am.

Many cultures had intermittent fasting figured out thousands of years ago. Sometimes it wasn't even a choice - they just didn't have regular access to food! We've been slower in the Western world to pick this up — eating to stimulate your metabolism is a load of rubbish. Eating six small regular meals a day is like telling an alcoholic to have just a few little drinks every day — it's a set up for disaster.

With 50% of society overweight or obese, we need to take a look at what we have been conditioned to believe is true and where this information came from. Many people are waking up and throwing down a breakfast meal on top of last night's dinner that the body has not yet metabolised.

It's not healthy and can lead to long-term ramifications for the gut, bowel and intestines. Give the digestive process a rest and let the body clean itself out. This process is called autophagy — it's like spring-cleaning for our dead cells — and it happens when we fast.

There are a few different versions of intermittent fasting; however, this one, with the eight-hour eating window and 16-hour fasting window, seems to be the most practical. Lots of people find it easy to wake up, exercise, get ready for work, sort the kids out, and do whatever else they have to do without worrying about finding time to eat. When the day has settled into a routine, the idea is to eat two to three meals between midday and 8 pm.

Morning fasting is also the ultimate compensation strategy for times when you overeat at dinner, have a few drinks, or eat late. It can all be counteracted by making your first meal the next day at midday or later.

During the morning, the hunger might come in waves that last five to ten minutes — just ignore them and associate those feelings with better health. If you are new to this, the first couple of days will be the hardest but after a while, you will wonder why you were worrying about eating a meal first thing in the day for the last 30 years.

If you need a new mantra, you can tell yourself that breakfast is the most important meal of the day … to skip. It is not just good for weight loss — it is terrific for overall health.

How to Stay Motivated

WOW, I really regret
that workout.

- No One Ever

Your health — is there anything more important?

Your health and the way you look both feed into one another and influence the way you feel about yourself.

They influence your confidence and self-esteem — and that's what I really care about. The deeper emotions! And not dying early in life is beneficial too.

It's about poor health not negatively affecting your quality of life. I see people in their 40s and 50s who are so immobile they can't reach down to tie their shoes, or who take 60 seconds to stand up from laying down on the floor.

That's not awesome, and it won't rectify itself without a concerted effort.

The people I meet want to lose weight, be healthier and have more vitality. Achieving this is about nutrition and exercise. Consistency. Routine. Habit.

One of the most pleasing aspects of my work is helping people who do not consider themselves to be a 'gym person' or an 'exercise person' and then seeing them establish a consistent, enjoyable routine and actually fall in love with exercise.

In many cases, the issue is not that the individual was never motivated — they just weren't sure what to do or where to start. Maybe they were intimidated by going to a big gym.

Maybe they lacked confidence in themselves. Or perhaps they'd tried an exercise routine at some point in the past and didn't stick with it, didn't seem to get the results they were looking for or found it boring.

I often like to use the example of an athlete in cases like this. Athletes are never 'on' for 52 weeks per year. They have an on-season, an off-season and a pre-season.

The off-season is where they might relax and refresh, the pre-season is where the focus restarts, and the on-season is a purpose-driven period focused on results.

We can think of ourselves the same way. Sometimes we are in the zone and sometimes we relax and loosen up. The idea is to be in a good routine more often than not. Sometimes we just go through the motions and that's alright. I always say it's better to exercise and eat crap than to not exercise and eat crap.

Is it possible to go from not being motivated to being motivated?

It certainly is!

Modelling Success

In my research for this chapter, I spoke to some clients and other people I've known for a long time. I spoke with people who had lost 40 kilograms, regained it, lost it again — and then kept it off. I spoke to people who have exercised consistently since childhood, and to people who took up exercise in their 50's and have been doing remarkably well with it for the last ten years.

The people who are difficult to get feedback from are those who exercise for a few months, then have a few years off.

Back to the people who are doing well with their exercise, nutrition and weight management. Two key words kept popping up when I was talking to them — routine and habit. For this reason, I've zeroed in on the notion of developing a consistent routine as a crucial component in maintaining motivation.

There's a book called Atomic Habits, written by James Clear. The book looks at common themes and habits among successful people. Clear says that when you identify those, you should do the same things yourself in order to establish the same methods for success in your own life.

Anthony Robbins also has a concept called 'modelling'. He says you just need to find someone who succeeded in doing what you are trying to do, and do what they did. So let's apply this to exercise.

Commonalities among people who achieve long-term success with their exercise:

- Putting their exercise sessions in their weekly schedule first, not last. The rest of their life fits in around their exercise
- They exercise daily. People eventually find it's easier to do something daily, than it is to do it three times a week
- They exercise whether they feel like it or not. It is not always about performing your best – it's about turning up, doing it and keeping the routine going

- People who exercise frequently tend to make healthier food choices. When people don't exercise, they place less emphasis on quality nutrition
- People who are successful with their exercise and have great energy levels often do not eat before 11am each day

How will these points help you stay motivated? The answer — they lead to incredible results. That's motivating! They also make realistic guidelines for establishing a lifelong exercise routine or habit.

When you're creating an exercise routine, you need to create a plan and a strategy. Look at your week. Look at the timetable of your gym. Think about your work and family commitments.

Now, stick all your exercise into your calendar FIRST!

Lots of people plan their week and put exercise in later. The result?

Exercise doesn't always happen this way. Once your exercise sessions are locked into your weekly schedule, just do them — whether you feel like it or not. It's not about performing well when you exercise. It's about simply doing it.

Sometimes people say, "Oh, I didn't do as well as normal today". Who cares? You did it! That's amazing!

There's a popular saying: "90% of success is turning up". Just turn up. Even if you go through the motions. I have lost count of the number of times someone has come to training feeling like crap and left feeling amazing. It's not just the physical feeling that makes you feel good; it's the self-pride, which you are completely entitled to, that makes you feel happy with yourself.

Half of my work is with people who love exercise — it is so important to them that they can't NOT do it. In fact, they need more discipline to have a day off exercising than they need to come and train. The other half of my work is with people who know they should exercise; however, it doesn't come naturally to them.

They benefit from support and encouragement. I love working with both categories of people. I think it is valuable to be aware of which group you fall into so you can surround yourself with the right people, tools and resources for success.

Change

One massive topic in my line of work is CHANGE. Change is hard. People often seek support, coaching and accountability when the pain of remaining the same becomes greater than the pain involved with making a change.

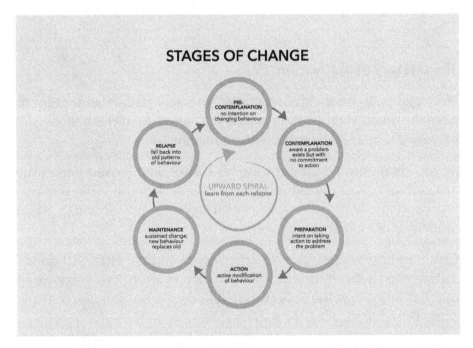

In a health-coaching relationship, change does not happen overnight. Often, I have to build a relationship, foster trust, and instil a sense of self-belief in people, before more positive habits become ingrained.

I understand that leading an active lifestyle and making healthy food choices comes naturally to some people but not to everyone.

People have to be met where they are. This, combined with the fact that a one-size-fits-all approach does not work, is something I love about my vocation.

As a young personal trainer, 20 years ago, I learnt very quickly that reprimanding people or making them feel bad about eating unhealthy food does not work nearly as well as support and encouragement. In saying that, a coach needs to be motivated too.

Nobody wants to spend their days with an energy vampire. If a significant amount of time passes without a certain level of results being achieved, it could be time to move on — for the sake of the client and the coach. It has to be a partnership — with both parties being motivated and committed.

The Mystery of Motivation

Motivation can be tricky. Sometimes, the very people who seem to have the greatest motivation just don't change. Martin is a successful 48-year-old real estate agent with young children.

At 150 kilograms, he sat opposite his doctor who looked him in the eye and said, "You will die soon if you remain like this". That was two years ago, and Martin is now heavier. A life of physical abundance and mobility looks extremely unlikely.

Catherine and her son have an extremely rare blood type. Catherine's son required a kidney donor. After exhausting all options, it appeared that Catherine was the only compatible donor, but she was told she could only donate a kidney if she lost 30 kilograms.

Two years later, Catherine has not lost one kilogram, and her son still needs a kidney.

What's going on in these two stories?

It is not a lack of education. Martin and Catherine could not have had more compelling reasons to get healthy. This brings me back to my point that motivation is very tricky. It's not cut and dry for everyone.

Let's look at two positive, inspiring examples of people who were able to seize on powerful ways to get motivated and stay that way.

Paul's Motivation to Change: An Epiphany

I coached Paul — an amazing man. He's 52 years old, runs a successful international company, has a great social life and is a devoted father.

Paul struggled to exercise consistently for three decades, between the ages of 20 and 50. He said that one day, he woke up and had an epiphany: for 30 years, he had treated exercise like it was optional. He would wake up and ask himself, "Will I exercise today?"

At the age of 50, he said he stopped treating exercise like it was optional and made it part of each day. I met Paul in 2011, and he has exercised six times a week since then and continues to do so.

The thing is, for three years, Paul said his goal was weight loss, but despite going to the gym six times a week, he never lost a kilo. He said he was not willing to give up two glasses of wine each night, or dining out, or toast with his eggs each morning.

With a high level of emotional intelligence, Paul could engage in a deep conversation about the fact his behaviour with food wasn't in line with his goals. Upon reflection, he came to the realisation that his goal was not actually weight loss but increasing his fitness and enjoying the mental benefits to be experienced from exercising daily.

Paul went on to run a marathon and he travels the world, skiing. He still drinks wine, guilt-free!

Troy's Motivation to Change: Results

I've mentioned Troy previously, but his story serves many purposes, so I'll talk about him again. Troy never had a problem with exercise motivation. Back when we first met in 2002, he went from 127 kilograms to 110 kilograms over a period of a few years. But things happen and life gets in the way, and by 2016, he was back to around 136 kilograms again.

A few things happened in Troy's life, including a couple of health scares and the passing of a dear friend due to brain cancer. As we approach mid-life, we get a sense of our own mortality and, whether consciously or subconsciously, we start to shift our values.

In 2018, I suggested to Troy that he try intermittent fasting. This idea was met with some resistance. Still, he gave it a go — slowly starting by having his first meal at 9am, then 10am, then 11am.

Now, he flies through the morning on a couple of black coffees with a dash of milk, and his energy and mental acuity are better than ever.

On top of that, Troy now weighs 101 kilograms, which is the lightest he's been since high school. With his height and frame, he looks incredible right where he is now.

Troy still enjoys a beer and a paddle pop, but he has grasped the concept of being in a calorie deficit, the timing of his meals, burning fat, and a bunch of other things that make weight loss and living in peak health effortless and efficient.

The fact that you're not where you want to be should be enough motivation.

Motivation can come and go. I have lost count of the number of people I have met who have lost ten kilograms and regained the ten kilograms, or lost 20 kilograms and then found it again … multiple times!

When you achieve your weight loss goal, you need to think of that point as THE BEGINNING.

This is often when people need the most help – not when they back off and go into maintenance mode — which is a myth, by the way.

Most people call it THE END when they arrive at their goal weight. In the end, they stop, or back off. They become complacent and reintroduce poor food choices into their diet.

People with great bodies don't get to where they want to be and then relax. They place eating well and exercising every day in the same category as brushing their teeth, showering and breathing.

It's done daily with no thought to not doing it. It's not optional, and they don't want it to be.

**Long-term consistency
trumps short-term intensity.**

- Bruce Lee

The 80/20 Rule

Put simply, the 80/20 Rule tells us that 20% of our activities will account for 80% of our results.

It's a business concept that can be easily and successfully applied to any aspect of our life.

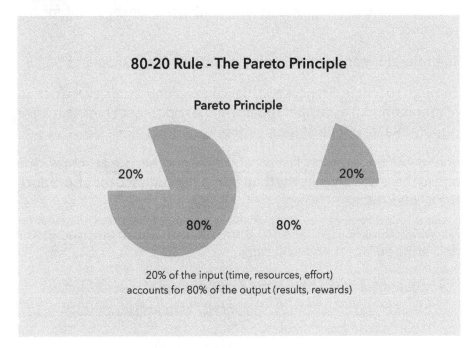

80-20 Rule - The Pareto Principle

Pareto Principle

20%

80%

20%

80%

20% of the input (time, resources, effort)
accounts for 80% of the output (results, rewards)

Who came up with this concept?

Vilfredo Federico Damaso Pareto was an Italian philosopher and economist, born in 1848. It is said he was inspired to think about the uneven distribution of wealth and production, based on an observation of the generation of pea pods in his garden.

The figures he came up with were 80% and 20%, leading to the generalisation that 80% of results arise from a mere 20% of the action.

How does this principle apply to exercise and nutrition?

I am a big fan of efficiency. I like to ask my clients, "What are the 20% of things you can do that will be responsible for 80% of your results?"

For Karen, it was eating her meals between midday and 8 pm (intermittent fasting) and exercising five times per week. The morning fast reduced her daily calorie intake and was the ultimate compensation strategy for any time she didn't eat perfectly; and she found the exercise easier than the nutrition plan, as most people do. Karen lost 12 kilograms in six months and looked great for her wedding.

Then she stopped personal training and gained six kilograms.

Through coaching, Jayne has achieved excellent results over a period of four months. I asked her to tell me the top three things that were responsible for her outstanding progress.

She identified morning fasting and reducing her sugar intake. She added there wasn't really the third thing, although she did also reduce her alcohol intake.

For most people I work with, the two most important things for delivering 80% of their results are:

- eating all meals between 12 pm and 8 pm
- exercising consistently, specifically with resistance training as part of the exercise plan.

Other things that make a massive impact on helping you achieve peak health include:

- reducing sugar
- reducing or eliminating alcohol

- not snacking
- removing milky coffees from your diet
- exercising four times a week
- having your measurements taken each month.

Everyone has two or three things they can focus on (their 20%) that will unlock the door to massive results (their 80%). What are yours?

inLove

SCOTT CAPELIN

Your Relationship With Yourself

> It is only when you have mastered
> the art of loving yourself that you can
> truly love others. It's only when you have
> opened your own heart that you can
> touch the hearts of others. When you feel
> centered and alive, you are in much
> better position to be a better person.
>
> - Robin Sharma

It's hard to be in top shape if you don't like who you are. I've seen plenty of people attempt to 'hate themselves all the way to skinny', and it's a tough road.

It is challenging to live the life of your dreams when you don't feel worthy. It is difficult to be your best if you don't have a positive network of people supporting and encouraging you.

If you are in an intimate relationship, it's a great investment of your time and energy to make it the best it can be. You cannot attract positive when you are thinking and feeling negative.

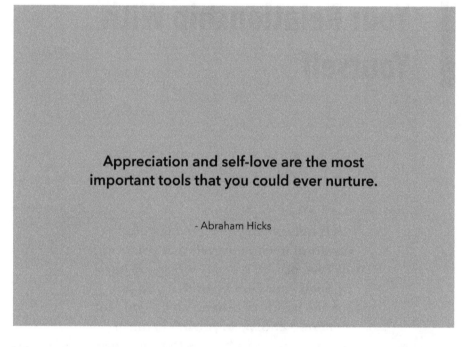

Appreciation and self-love are the most important tools that you could ever nurture.

- Abraham Hicks

When you are in great shape, you have the enthusiasm to do more of the things you love, and the energy to pursue a life of inspiration.

When you are in love with your life and have a great relationship with yourself, it provides the self-confidence to take control of your health, and the spark to live an inspired life of passion and purpose.

And when you feel inspired, you have the drive to be in peak shape and the desire to live a life you love!

If you don't have a great relationship with yourself, it could be argued that you are no good to anyone. First and foremost, it is your responsibility to become the very best person you can be. From there, your own life will be filled with a greater level of abundance, joy and beauty. You will exude an aura that has a positive effect on those people closest to you.

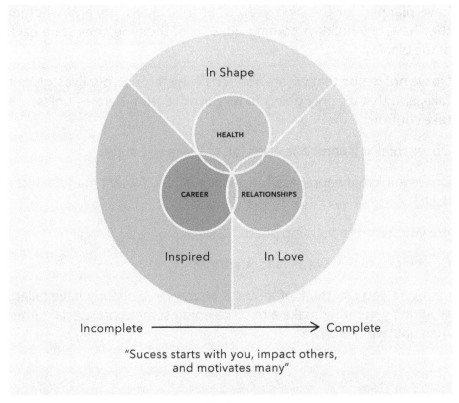

In Shape

HEALTH

CAREER   RELATIONSHIPS

Inspired   In Love

Incomplete ⟶ Complete

"Sucess starts with you, impact others,
and motivates many"

We have seven times more conversations with ourselves, through our internal dialogue, than we do with everyone else in our life combined.

The way we speak to ourselves, and in turn, think and feel about ourselves, has a monumental impact on our actions, behaviour and physiology, and ultimately, on the outcomes we produce for ourselves.

Whilst I love helping people achieve physical results in terms of strength, fitness, weight loss, and improved appearance, the main purpose behind my work is to improve the mental and emotional state of my clients. People often say, "I will feel happier and more confident when I lose ten kilograms". Let me tell you that, with a small mindset shift, you can be happier and more confident right now.

It really is not fair — to yourself or to others — to be dragging your butt through life, operating at 60% and being a drain on those around you. Whenever I speak to people who are flat, I ask them what they have planned for the next year, what their goals are, and whether they have any holidays coming up. 95% of the time, they stare back at me blankly.

Do we not realise that we are about halfway through our lives, give or take, and that it's only going to be downhill from here — unless we take control?

Do we think it is someone else's job to make us happy?

Do we think that happiness, satisfaction, and fulfilment manufactures itself?

Are you scared to set a big goal?

Do you realise that we all fail sometimes?

I am sure you can think of a bunch of ways you already have failed. Wouldn't you rather make a mistake doing something special rather than not trying at all?

To fall in love with yourself is the first secret to happiness

-Robert Morley

Abundance, joy and beauty live on the other side of fear, and way outside your comfort zone.

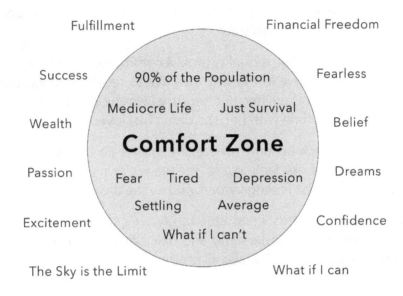

Relationships

This isn't a book offering relationship advice, however, if it was, there would be a few very basic criteria recommended to strengthen your intimate relationship.

There's a book called The Five Love Languages by Dr Gary Chapman. He says that there are five ways we can make someone feel loved, and each of us has one preferred way. The five love languages are:

- quality time
- words of affirmation
- receiving gifts
- acts of service
- physical touch.

The book is a great read, and not a lengthy one. However, if you're thinking, "I ain't got time to read another book!" do a search on

YouTube and watch a six-minute summary.

I credit this book for largely saving my marriage. My love language is 'words of affirmation'. Every now and then, it's nice for me to hear I'm doing well and am appreciated.

My wife's love language is 'quality time'. A common issue is that people generally express love in the way they like to receive it. I was telling Lauren how much I love her, but because I was working a lot and not spending quality time with her, she didn't feel loved.

And there was a long time where she wasn't an overly expressive communicator of her feelings, so she wasn't giving me the words I needed and I wasn't feeling valued, and so the divide grew.

Once I understood this, I was able to give her the time she needed and she was able to understand and deliver the things I needed to feel loved. As it turns out, it was all pretty easy and now I'm even a bit of a 'quality time' guy.

From the list above, do you know your partner's love language?

Do you know your partner's top five core values?

And do you respect them?

Do you feel you're on the same page in regard to your future plans and how you look at life?

And do you talk about this? Do you have shared goals?

The chances of two people growing together and looking at the world the same way for 50 years can be slim, but knowing the fundamentals helps maintain harmony and maximise understanding, respect and passion.

You need to carry your best self into your intimate relationship, into your parenting and into your work. It is irresponsible and negligent not to.

I have a big background in a team sport, and also working with teams of people in a business environment. I love teamwork.

Having a group of people who are on the same page, taking pride in working towards a worthy objective is one of the most fulfilling experiences you can have.

When it comes to your intimate relationship with your spouse or partner, I see that as a two-person team, and it's the most important team you will ever be on, so it makes sense to keep this team strong.

There's an American author by the name of Jackson Brown who wrote a bestseller called "Life's Little Instruction Book". He is well known for a famous quote that says "Marry the right person. This one decision will determine 90% of your happiness or misery."

That might be true, or it might not be true for you.

If you have a partner, it's probably too late now to go back and choose them, because you've already done that, so all you can focus on doing is making them the right person, and making your relationship as great as it can be. Or if it's not great you can leave.

You might think it's too hard and painful to leave, so you decide to stay in an unhappy relationship. And if that's you then you really do have two choices – to make a concerted effort to make your relationship the best it can possibly be, or move on.

Choosing to remain passive in an unfulfilling relationship isn't always the most noble option.

If I can proclaim to be any kind of authority on this topic it is for three reasons:

1. I have made pretty much every mistake a person can make in this area
2. I have spent a lifetime studying it
3. I am passionate about helping people

It goes back to the title of this book. I do believe we can be in excellent health, have satisfying and uplifting interpersonal relationships, and live a life of passion and purpose that inspires us. It's not that hard.

A Final Note on Relationships

I think of love like a game of tennis. This is a personal analogy and I hope it makes sense. Someone has to serve (and you are serving love).

When two givers indulge in a connection, it's alchemy. I water you, you water me, we never drain each other, we just grow.

Ideally, the serve is returned with a loving act, and when you return the act, and then it's hit back again, and so on. I call it Love Tennis. It makes sense to me. I have never really understood why the more love I give, the more I feel loved. It's almost like doing nice things for my wife isn't even about her – it just makes me feel good! Although it really is about her.

You can't have love going back and forth if nobody is hitting balls. Just keep swinging! People get resentful and stop expressing love.

Some people won't do loving acts for their partner because they feel like their partner doesn't deserve it or hasn't earned it. That's a road to nowhere. I would challenge you to make a list of things you can do to make your partner feel loved, and take action on this by implementing 2 items on your list every week for 4 weeks, and watch how the love is returned to you.

Choice, Challenge, and Change

Let's turn to Matt to see how it looks when someone makes the decision to carry their best self into all areas of life and to live life to the fullest. Here's his story:

It was December 2003, and I had been Matt's personal trainer for two years. In that time, we had become good friends. He had gone from 143 kilograms to 93 kilograms and had increased his self-confidence a great deal. Matt was 24 years old, and he had never had a girlfriend.

Then, he asked a young lady on a date, and she said yes. He turned up to our personal training that day with some other news too.

After a long period of deliberation, he had decided to leave his job as an accountant in one of the top firms in the city, to pursue his dream of entering the fitness industry.

A desire for weight loss was the catalyst for Matt to seek support and accountability to improve his life, but the ripple effect from achieving this goal filtered through to every other aspect of his life.

He ended up with a girlfriend who saw the very best in him, and a new job that he loved. It's results like this that have made me fall in love with my vocation.

Fast-forward 15 years — Matt is married to that woman and they have three beautiful children. His career has evolved and he's now a very successful business mentor. He exercises every week and has the balance he wants.

"Live life fully while you're here. Experience everything. Take care of yourself and your friends. Have fun, be crazy, be weird. Go out and screw up! You're going to anyway, so you might as well enjoy the process. Take the opportunity to learn from your mistakes: find the cause of your problem and eliminate it. Don't try to be perfect; just be an excellent example of being human."

-Tony Robbins

This all sounds great, but where do I start?

So how do you enhance your self-image?

How do you live a life of passion and purpose?

You do this by doing things that make you grow as a person and by doing things that are bigger than yourself. If you want more, you have to give more. By giving more, you receive more.

> **When we strive to become better than we are, everything around us becomes better, too.**
>
> -Paulo Coelho, The Alchemist

All the resources we need are available to us. All the help, time, money, people, knowledge and expertise are there, we just need to look for them and take action.

We need to believe it is all possible.

And we need to be mentally strong.

Setting goals that set your heart alight – goals both large and small – and achieving them, or even just coming close, is one of the surest ways to live a life of passion and purpose.

Personal growth is the by-product, meaning you become a better person in the process.

Many people say it is not even about the achievement of the goal; what makes the difference is the person you become in the process.

What kind of person do you want to be? Do you want to have that look in your eye that says you are on this planet for a reason and that every day, you are moving forward and going somewhere worthwhile?

> We do not believe in ourselves until
> someone reveals that deep inside us something
> is valuable, worth listening to, worthy of our trust,
> sacred to our touch. Once we believe in ourselves
> we can risk curiosity, wonder, spontaneous delight
> or any experience that reveals the human spirit.
>
> - E. E. Cummings

Or, will next year be like this year, which was like last year?

The X-Factor

Anthony Robbins says that when you see someone you find attractive, it is not their looks that are appealing but the sense of freedom that is most alluring.

They will have an aura and an X-Factor that is hard to define. To understand this better, think of someone you know who isn't free.

Are they attractive?

Are they attracting opportunities?

Do people want to be around them?

Do they seem trapped or stuck?

Could this be you?

Are you an energy vampire — or are you itching to jump out of bed each morning and attack the day?

There is a whole host of personal development tools out there, waiting for us to open our eyes and broaden our world. They come in the form of books, seminars, videos, coaches and mentors. Just one conversation can change your life. It's completely different from speaking with a friend or family member.

You need the unbiased, objective opinion of someone who is skilled in helping people get the most out of life. This was true for me. Let me share some stories of how I was able to change from living a decent and average life, to living with passion and zest.

In 2003, I had a personal training client who was in her 70's and who owned three pharmacies. We got along well. She always wanted to be pushed to the limit with her exercise and with her life.

She went overseas three times each year, did Tai-Chi every week and learned to play musical instruments. In her spare time, she would buy investment properties, make improvements to them and sell them.

She told me a story once about how her accountant asked her why she was doing so many things. He suggested that with the money she had, she could simply retire.

"RETIRE????" she yelled at him indignantly. "If I retire, I may as well be dead!"

Her accountant never made that suggestion again.

We got along well and she must have seen potential in me, which at that stage needed some harnessing. She purchased a $1,500 ticket to a four-day personal development seminar for me and encouraged me to go. I almost didn't attend. I'm glad I did. I really feel it changed my life.

My second story takes place in June 2004, when I was feeling some dissatisfaction with life. I was almost 28 years old, and I engaged in the services of a life coach.

We spoke in-depth, and I recall leaving our first session with three clear major goals:

1. Open my own business
2. Purchase a property
3. Enter into a fulfilling, deeply loving, intimate relationship

Within six months, I had achieved all three goals. This really opened my eyes to the power of coaching.

So, step one in positive change is the awareness that you need to love yourself and be proud of the person you are. Think about ways you can make this happen.

Create in your mind, a vision of the person you want to be and the life you want to live.

> We are all flesh and bones. We all come from the same universal source. However, the ones who do more than just exist, the ones who fan the flames of their human potential and truly savor the magical dance of life do different things than those whose lives are ordinary. Foremost among the things that they do is adopt a positive paradigm about their world and all that is in it.
>
> - Robin Sharma

Identifying Your Values

Values are a lens through which you see the world,
and they provide a filter for making
the right decisions.

- Scott Capelin

One thing I like to identify in myself and others when looking for reasons to explain behaviour is our personal core values. These may be loosely defined as the things that are most important to you in your life.

Take a look at some of the major values you might have in your life: family, finances, health, career, relationships, travel, social life, or any other topic you feel most compelled to dedicate your time to.

Values and standards are closely related. When someone isn't performing, or their behaviour doesn't align with the goals they have stated, I ask them to think about their values.

Perhaps the goals we have set aren't in line with their values and maybe that's why they're not feeling driven to achieve them? On occasion, I'll ask people to think about their standards, and whether any of their standards, in certain areas of life, are lower for some reason.

Do areas of low standards indicate low values?

And what does it mean if you want to be in shape but you eat some form of junk food every single day?

What does it mean if someone is super successful at their work, if they are an amazing mother, or if they volunteer to help less fortunate people three times a week, yet they can't establish and maintain a routine with exercise and nutrition?

Does it mean they are a failure, lazy or a bad person? Certainly not!

Does it mean that health and fitness aren't important to them and are not among their top values?

Maybe it does. I know that when I tell myself I should do something, and six months later I haven't done it, I can usually stop, analyse the situation and see it's actually not that important to me.

It's not aligned with one of my top values, so that's why I didn't change my behaviour and do it.

Personal and professional development expert, Dr John Demartini, says, "Your voids drive your values". A void is where something is missing from your life. A value is something you desire. So, it makes sense that you might want something you don't have because you believe your life will be better if you have it.

This is a void.

Here's an example of what can happen when you have an unfulfilled void.

First, you might get a food craving to subconsciously fill the void. This may then lead to health issues, such as excess weight, lethargy or skin irritation. These are all emotional issues manifesting physically.

Third, illness and disease follow. The food cravings show up first, but, make no mistake, illness and disease will come. It may take five, ten or 20 years but it will hit you and hit you hard. That's why I take all of this so seriously.

Why would a void result in overeating?

We all have needs that must be met. If they are not met one way, our psyche will find another way to meet them. What are these needs?

The image below shows Tony Robbins' Six Human Needs model.

SIX HUMAN NEEDS:
- Certainty
- Variety
- Significance
- Love/Connection
- Growth
- Contribution

Certainty

We need to know where we will sleep tonight, who loves us, how much money we have in the bank, where the next lot of money will come from, and where our next meal is coming from. Imagine what it would be like not knowing these things?

Variety

Ironically, variety is also uncertainty, which is the opposite of the value outlined above. When things are boring or there's too much of the same, too often, we look for something different.

When I was quite young, I was in a personal development seminar and the speaker said, "When someone has no uncertainty in their life, watch them create some drama".

Love and Connection

As we move through the list these human needs become deeper. Love and connection is a big one, and many people connect with food. It also meets the need for certainty because we know the food will taste great and make us feel good – albeit temporarily.

And, in terms of variety, the amount of food a person can binge on is endless. We also need love from other people, and we have a need to connect, which could be with people, or with your work. A lack of connection to your core values in the work you do will result in job dissatisfaction.

Significance

A person who doesn't feel significant or connected to their partner will find a way to meet these needs elsewhere, possibly via work, or with another person. Significance can be derived from being a parent, throwing yourself into your career or coaching the local soccer team.

Growth and Contribution

These final two needs are referred to as 'Higher Needs'. I speak a lot about growth because it's essential for our self-actualisation – becoming the best you can be. It is the ultimate aim in Maslow's Hierarchy of Needs (see the next diagram), along with contribution.

For a long time I never fully understood contribution.

Why does James Packer keep working when he has enough money for ten lifetimes?

Clearly, his work meets many of the Six Human Needs.

Why would a busy person volunteer to coach the local netball team?

Why is becoming a parent such an inherent need?

All these things we do, the extras, fulfil our need to contribute to a cause greater than ourselves.

A lack of contribution can lead to a lack of purpose, which can then lead to those voids being filled with other things that aren't so positive.

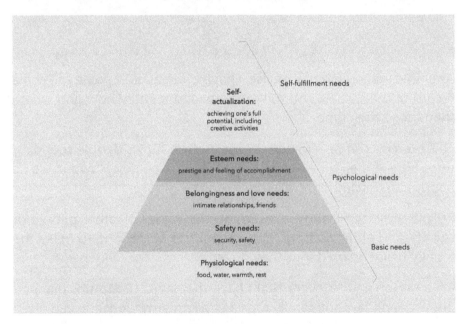

The key to having a life you love is to have an intimate understanding of your most important core personal values as a human being and then live a life that is aligned with those values.

The reason for this is that we all find time for the things that are important to us according to our values. Most unhappiness stems from living a life that is not in accordance with our values.

> **Values determine behaviour.**
> **Standards dictate results.**
>
> - Scott Capelin

As a time management exercise, I have often asked people to keep a record of their week, and their month, and identify how and where they spend their time.

This exercise can be eye-opening as it often shows people spending up to 80% of their time doing things they don't enjoy. How can we be happy and fulfilled living like this?

People are often living according to the values of other people or society, and either waiting for the weekend or working to make the money to spend on things they do enjoy.

On a personal note, every year I have the entire 12 months planned out with holidays and family trips away. I love my work and can often become immersed in it, working long hours.

The best way for me to create balance and ensure I live in line with my 'family' values, is to book weekends away each month, and longer holidays four times each year. I also structure my work hours so they are as efficient as possible and allow for time with family, and time to exercise for a couple of hours each day.

The steps to living a life of passion and inspiration can be identified as follows:

- Identify your highest priority values
- Set goals in line with these values
- Create a visual and written description of what this all looks like
- Take steps to bring it all to fruition

(This process is outlined in more detail later in the book.)

Identifying Your Values

Are you are wondering how you can identify your values? This is how I identified mine.

It was March 2015, and I had been married to Lauren for seven years. We had one daughter and another on the way – our lives had changed a lot since the days of no children.

The pressures of our work had increased. I was looking for a solution to improve our marriage and also seeking answers to the lack of fulfilment I was feeling with my life overall.

I booked myself into a seven-day, personal development seminar on the other side of the country. There were about 50 people at the seminar. On the fourth day, we were asked to undertake a written exercise.

At the top of the page were these instructions: *You have two years to live. Between now and that time, you are in perfect health. How will you spend your time?*

Overcome with inspiration, I grabbed my pen. The words flowed out of my mind and onto the page without me even having to think. I described the way I would travel the world with my wife and children, and how I would experience all the beauty this world has to offer. I described, in detail, how Lauren and I would invite our mothers along so we could spend time with them, and so they could also be with us and our kids – and help us with the kids!

The entire two years would be a period of quality family time and adventure! I listed all the countries we would visit and described how we would have the greatest time doing exciting things, and also spend time relaxing and doing nothing at all.

We would experience freedom at its finest and be grateful for it every day.

Now, you have to realise that, at the time, I was heavily focused on my business pursuits. This contributed to the distance in my marriage. I was also extremely focused on my physical training. As an example, I brought my own food — fish, salad, chicken and vegetables — to the seminar because I was just a few weeks out from participating in a bodybuilding competition.

The guy who was running the seminar was pretty incredible, and he was also super blunt and direct. I had just finished writing my response to what I would do with my final two years on this planet, when he walked right up to me, pulled out his red pen, read my notes and circled three words:

- family
- freedom
- travel

He looked me in the eye and said, "These are your top values?"

I said, "No, they're not. You don't know me. My top values are business and exercise".

He asked me whether I would go to work every day and go to the gym every day if I had just two years to live. I said no.

He said, "Well, they aren't your top values then".

A massive wave of emotion washed over me and in front of the whole seminar group I burst out crying. No wonder I had felt so off-track. I was living a life that didn't match my primary values.

The seminar facilitator didn't bat an eyelid. He looked at me and asked, "What are you crying for?"

I said, "I've been such an idiot!"

He explained to me that I wasn't an idiot, but I had been living in a way that I thought was important, by doing things that may have supported my main values. For example, having a successful business could give me the money I needed to travel and look after my family, and since most of my business pursuits were in the health and fitness sector, it supported my career to be in good shape.

However, the crucial pieces of the puzzle I was missing were: why I was doing what I was doing, and how to be able to best communicate that to the people I was doing it for.

More importantly, now that I had clarity regarding my values, I could spend my time and energy with my family, taking holidays and creating a work structure that allowed me freedom, rather than doing it all the wrong way around, like I was, up to that point.

Shortly after that, Lauren and I flew to Fiji to renew our wedding vows, and our marriage has been about as close to perfect as it can get since then.

Since that time, over the years, I have studied and analysed my personal values in more depth. Here is my current list:

- gratitude
- fun
- happiness
- family
- growth
- freedom
- finances

- faith
- adventure
- business
- contribution
- travel
- health
- inspiration

> This is a call to all you sleepin' souls
> Wake up and take control of your own cipher
> And be on the lookout for the spirit snipers
> Tryin' to steal your light, you know
> what I'm sayin'?
> Look within-side yourself, for peace
> Give thanks, live life and release
> You dig me? You got me?
>
> - Public Enemy (He Got Game)

Other Ways to Determine Your Values

Values can be an activity or a quality. For example, some people value honesty, which is a quality. Some people love to run marathons, which is an activity.

There aren't too many rules in terms of identifying what you value the most!

A value is anything that is important to you. Choose whatever you like — they're your values.

Here are a few ways you could identify your values:

1. Ask yourself the following questions to explore the values that are most important to you.

- What do you never have to be reminded to do?
- How do you spend most of your time?
- What do you think about the most?
- Where do you spend your money?
- In the space where you live and work, what clues are there that point to your values?

2. Google 'list of core values' and choose the ones that resonate with you.

3. Think about these scenarios:

- You have two years to live but you still have to go to work and you can't go crazy maxing out credit cards – what do you do? Increase the urgency by making it six months to live.
- You're going to die tomorrow. What will you do between now and then? Most people say they will call people and tell them they love them, the thing is – you should be doing this now.
- You're going to die tomorrow, however, an angel comes to you and says you can have an extra 40 years to live under two conditions:
  1. You have to do work you are passionate about.
  2. Your work must contribute positively to society.

So, what work will you choose to do?

Once again, you are going to experience a lot more fulfilment in your life if you start doing that now. Live in alignment with those values now. Start doing that kind of work now.

The average retirement age is 67 years old. The average age of death is 78. Are you going to wait until you're 67 to have 11 years of life?

If you live by your own hierarchy of values, you'll thrive. If you live by someone else's values or society's values, you die a little inside each day.

Many people are driving a car they can't afford to a job they don't like, to pay for the car they can't afford.

They spend so much time in their stressful job which impacts or eliminates time they could be spending with family and friends, or exercising, or just having fun.

Values are Intensely Personal

Most arguments start because two people are looking at the same situation through different perspectives. It's a clash of values. One of the number one guidelines for happiness and inner peace is the awareness that we cannot control what anyone else says, does or thinks, so don't bother wasting energy on the values, choices, and decisions other people make.

Another very similar rule for happiness is that we can only focus on what we can control.

Why get upset about the weather, or who won the election, if we can't control it?

A big key to peace and happiness in life is knowing what is worth worrying about, and what not to worry about. So often people get caught up in stuff that seriously doesn't matter. There's an old adage that says "If it's not going to matter in five years, don't worry about it for 5 seconds".

The truth is that not much of what's happening now will matter in 5 years, so if we lived by this philosophy we would be a lot less tense!

I am an NLP (Neuro-Linguistic Programming) Practitioner. A large part of NLP focuses on learning how to think and communicate more effectively with yourself and others.

There's a tool called the NLP Communication Model, seen in the image below.

NLP Communication Model

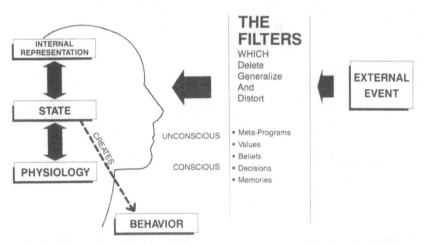

The model shows how a single event can turn into human behaviour. Basically, we experience an event that gets sent through a filter to be interpreted by our values and memories. A representation of the meaning of the event is created which ultimately determines our mood or state – and eventually our behaviour.

There are trillions of variables here, and the one thing I take away from it, is there is no way any two people on the planet can look at the same situation the same way.

Moral of the story: don't ever waste too much energy trying to change someone else's opinion of something.

> **God, give us grace to accept with serenity the things that cannot be changed, courage to change the things which should be changed and the wisdom to distinguish the one from the other.**
>
> - Reinhold Niebuhr

Two Tales: Christie and Ivan

Christie, a health coaching client, was a beautiful soul, smart, fun and bubbly. She had grown up in a loving family. Both her parents were accountants and encouraged Christie to become an accountant and work in the family business, guaranteeing her financial security.

Christie completed high school and achieved excellent exam results because she was a bright student. She went to university and became an accountant. She hated accounting. Most of our personal training sessions were spent exercising, rather uncomfortably given her overweight physical condition.

Christie had turned to food for comfort, to fill the void in her life and mask the lack of fulfilment she felt. She deeply wanted to become an artist ... something she is still yet to do.

What can we learn from Christie's plight?

Do you feel that open, honest communication with her parents would have helped? Would they have understood? Her parents felt they were doing what was best for her and Christie kept quiet because she didn't want to upset them.

Although it's hard to have those challenging conversations, only good things come from them. At the very least, Christie could have unburdened her pain, and even if nothing changed she wouldn't have been worse off!

The best-case scenario would be her parents thanking her for her candour and encouraging and supporting her in a change.

A lot of parents will do anything for their kids except let them be themselves.

This chapter finishes with a story from a book called *The Death of Ivan Ilyich*. It was written in 1886 by Leo Tolstoy. Most know Tolstoy from his classics, *War and Peace and Anna Karenina*. However, *The Death of Ivan Ilyich* contains poignant moments in relation to values that we can all learn from.

In the story, Ivan Ilyich spends his life climbing the social ladder and pursuing his legal career, mainly to immerse himself in something he can control, to make up for the unhappiness he feels within his marriage. As the title suggests, he does not have long to live, and a large part of the book deals with him reflecting upon the life he has lived and identifying it as an artificial life rather than an authentic life.

The story reaches its peak as Ivan lies on his death bed. Whilst holding the hand of his lifelong friend and colleague, he looks up and says, "What if my whole life has been wrong?"

Success, as judged by society, can often come at a great moral cost. As the book illustrates, this results in a life that is hollow and insincere, and, therefore, worse than death.

Don't be like Ivan.

Over the last 20 years, I have been in a front-row seat and seen up close, many wealthy, yet unhappy, people. Nobody teaches us how to be fulfilled, but it doesn't have to boil down to luck. We can plan and create our dream life and build perfect days. This is something we cover later in this book.

Action Item

The following two questions come from the author, Steve Siebold, who is one of the world's foremost experts in the field of critical thinking and mental toughness training.

Contemplate your responses to the following questions for a moment:

- If I could achieve a single thing in life, what would make all my hard work worth the struggle?
- If I had 30 seconds left to live, from what I've learned in life, what are the three most important things I would tell my children about how to live a happy life?

Your answers will tell you a lot about what drives you emotionally.

It is not your role to make others happy; it is your role to keep yourself in balance. When you pay attention to how you feel and practice self-empowering thoughts that align with who-you-really-are, you will offer an example of thriving that will be of tremendous value to those who have the benefit of observing you. You cannot get poor enough to help poor people thrive or sick enough to help sick peole get well. You only ever uplift from your position of strength and clarity and alignment.

-Abraham Hicks

The basis of your life is freedom, the purpose of your life is joy.

- Abraham Hicks

Success Leaves Clues

A giant ship's engine failed. The ship's owners tried one expert after another, but none of them could figure out how to fix the engine.

Then they brought in an old man who had been fixing ships since he was young.

He carried a large bag of tools with him and when he arrived, he immediately went to work. He inspected the engine very carefully, top to bottom.

Two of the ship's owners were there, watching this man, hoping he would know what to do.

After looking things over, the old man reached into his bag and pulled out a small hammer. He gently tapped something. Instantly, the engine lurched into life. He carefully put his hammer away. The engine was fixed.

A week later, the owners received a bill from the old man for $10,000. "What?" the owners exclaimed, "He hardly did anything!" So they wrote the old man a note, saying: Please send us an itemized bill.

The man sent a bill that read:

    Tapping with a hammer .... $ 2.00

    Knowing where to tap .... $ 9,998.00

This story highlights efficiency and experience. When it comes to optimising your health and relationships, and living a life of purpose and passion, it's like manipulating the tumblers on a safe.

Just a few tweaks in the right direction can unlock the door to enormous riches in terms of fulfilment, happiness, joy, beauty and abundance.

To use another analogy, most people aren't putting any thought or planning into these areas of their lives, which makes it more like pulling the lever on a poker machine and hoping they all align.

With that strategy, you have about as much chance of hitting the life fulfillment jackpot as you do of winning big in a casino.

I love the saying, "Success leaves clues". In order to achieve something, it's useful to look at people who have achieved what you want to do and find out what they did. I know a lot of people who live life *inShape inLove inSpired!* Here are common themes:

- They exercise just about every day
- If they fall off the wagon with exercise or nutrition, they get back on track quickly
- They eat light
- They don't obsess about their body
- They don't achieve their goal weight and then relax or see it as an endpoint
- They have mental resilience
- They live in a state of gratitude and appreciation
- They are surrounded by positive relationships and people who they support, and who support them in return
- They do work they love and have hobbies and interests they are passionate about
- They cut loose anyone who is not a positive influence on their life
- They understand their core personal values and live their life in line with them
- They have goals and a purpose that is bigger than just themselves
- They rarely complain

- They seek accountability

We don't need to reinvent the wheel. We just need to identify people who have succeeded at what we want to achieve and do what they did. If you find someone like that, ask them if you can catch up with them and ask for some advice.

I guarantee they will say yes, because contribution is one of the highest basic human needs, and it is prevalent in successful people.

SCOTT CAPELIN

Who Is Influencing You and How Are You Influencing Yourself?

**Whatever you are not changing
you are not choosing.**

Read that again.

There's an old quote that says: "You are the average of the five people you spend the most time with".

Have a think about who these people are for you.

Do they lift you up?

Do they make you a better person?

Do they support your ideas and goals?

Do they make you want to raise your standards?

Many people want you to go where they are going, which is nowhere. Hang around people who lift you up and support you; not people who crush or question your dreams.

These five people are referred to as your 'circle of influence' and it has been said that they can be responsible for up to 95% of your success, failure, happiness and fulfilment in life. It's fair to say they are pretty important.

Strive to surround yourself with positive, like-minded people who inspire you. To do that, you need to be a source of inspiration yourself.

> **Be careful whom you associate with. It is human to imitate the habits of those with whom we interact. We inadvertently adopt their interests, their opinions, their values, and their habit of of interpreting events.**
>
> -Epictetus

It can be challenging when we have had relationships for many years that we feel we have outgrown. We want to move onwards and upwards, but feel we are being held back.

In these cases, some open, honest conversations need to be had. In some instances, we need to untie the rope and move on from certain relationships if they aren't supporting the life we want to live.

Quite often, people drag you down from trying to get more out of life, because your growth and success make them feel inadequate about their lack of personal development. Trying to get you to remain at their level makes them feel comfortable and not as much of a failure.

Don't let anyone kill your vibe. If you have goals and dreams, people will point out the challenges and tell you things can't be done. This is a manifestation-killer. If you do dream big, most of the time you are better off not telling anyone about your aspirations. Only tell people that you know will support and encourage you, and better still, keep you accountable.

**Great minds discuss ideas,
average minds discuss events,
small minds discuss people.**

- Eleanor Roosevelt

> **We buy things we don't need with money**
> **we don't have to impress people we don't like.**
>
> - Dave Ramsey

Goals

Away from our external influences, we need to take time to think about our goals and how we want our days to be, and then create a vision of a life we will love.

The best ways to do this are:

- set goals for the next three months, 12 months, and three years in all the major areas of life
- write down a vision for your life
- create a dream board.

Just on 'goals' – personally, I believe I have achieved around 50% of the goals I've set for myself over the last two decades – which is pretty low for a driven person. On the other hand, during that time, I have achieved some incredible things that I didn't even set as a goal.

Does this make you wonder if there is any point in goal-setting at all?

With that in mind, let's not get hung up on the word 'goals'. Call them intentions and let them act as a compass to drive you in a particular direction. As Wayne Dyer says, "Be open to everything and attached to nothing".

Take a moment to think about your intentions.

Don't overthink it!

Create three columns – three-month intentions, 12-month intentions, three-year intentions – and jot down your responses to the following sections in each column:

Intention (goal) Setting

- health
- work
- relationship
- family
- friends
- financial
- social life
- personal growth

Note that your three-year intentions can be a bit looser – who knows what will be happening in three years? Have fun with this one!

In *The Surrender Experiment*, author, Michael Singer, spent a lifetime going where life's events took him and trusting there was a method behind the madness.

He proved there was. He says: "Life isn't about what we want, like or prefer, but the universe has a much higher plan for us than we could possibly be aware of".

This ties into another belief that helps me: "We don't have all the information". They say everything happens for a reason, but that provides no solace when you're going through a hard time and at that point, you don't know the reason.

Can you look back on your life now and see that the harsh relationship break-up allowed you to meet the love of your life?

Or how that job loss steered you towards a better opportunity?

Or, at the very least, how the things you learned through challenging experiences have increased your fortitude and mental strength, better equipping you for future problems?

Mark Manson says: "Life is a series of problems, and happiness actually comes from finding solutions. It's not that there will never be problems, but we can upgrade them to be better problems".

If you want to make God laugh, tell him about your plans.

- Woody Allen

Creating A Vision for Your Life

This is a visualisation exercise where the end result is a clear, inspiring written statement outlining exactly how you want your life to be.

Write it in the first person (I, me, my) and in the present tense. The idea is to read it regularly. Because your subconscious mind does not know the difference between fiction and reality, this vision becomes embedded in your subconscious, so over time, the universe will bring it all to fruition.

The easiest way to do this is a three-step process where, once again, you identify the most important areas of your life, and then do the following:

1. Write down what you **don't** want in these areas.
2. Reverse it all and write down what you **do** want.
3. Turn it into a story.

Here's an example:

Step 1— What I Don't Want

HEALTH: I don't want to be overweight and lacking energy. I don't want to struggle with the motivation to exercise. I don't want to be inconsistent with my training. I don't want to eat bad food.

WORK: I don't want a job I am bored in. I don't want to be checking my watch and hanging out for the weekend. I don't want to work in a negative environment.

RELATIONSHIP: I don't want to stay in a comfort zone. I don't want to lose the intimacy and excitement in my relationship. I don't want to fight with my partner.

FAMILY: I don't want to be distant from my family. I don't want any family divisions. I don't want my kids to feel less loved because I work long hours.

FRIENDS: I don't want to never go out and have fun. I don't want my long-term friendships to ever lose their magic.

FINANCIAL: I don't want to struggle with money and be living week to week. I don't want to be stressed about money.

SOCIAL LIFE: I don't want to ever go a year without an amazing holiday. I don't want to get lazy and not plan in advance for fun times with my friends.

PERSONAL GROWTH: I don't want to be bored or stuck in a rut. I don't want to be so busy and tired that I have no time to read or do further study.

Now you're ready for the next step – reverse every phrase to come up with something inspiring.

Step 2 — What I Do Want

HEALTH: I want to be lean, slim, fit, strong and athletic. I want to jump out of my skin with energy. I want to love my exercise and eat healthy, nutritious foods.

WORK: I love my work. The time flies because I am doing work I am passionate about. I want to work with people who are fun and inspiring, who make every day a pleasure!

RELATIONSHIP: I want to feel loved and love my partner deeply in return. I want to always make the effort to look great and plan dates and have fun. I want a partner who is my best friend and my favourite person in the world. I want someone I can communicate clearly with, and I want us to rarely have arguments, and if we do, we get over them quickly.

FAMILY: I want to be close to my family. I want a family who is loving and always there for one another. I want to spend quality time with my kids, so they can feel the love I have for them.

FRIENDS: I want to see my friends regularly. I want amazing friendships that last a lifetime.

FINANCIAL: I want to be a great saver of money and have money flow freely to me from multiple sources. I want to feel great about my financial position.

SOCIAL LIFE: I want to always have holidays booked to look forward to. I want to have days out and nights out. My life is filled with fun and adventure!

PERSONAL GROWTH: I want to always be growing and learning. I want to be stimulated by my ongoing levels of personal development.

Finally, the fun part – the finished product. Watch how everything from Step 2 is turned into a present tense narrative written in the first person.

Step 3 – Turn it Into a Story

I am lean, slim, fit, strong and athletic. I am a machine. I jump out of my skin every day with energy! I love my exercise, I train daily and I crave natural, healthy, nutritious foods. I love my work. I work with amazing people who make every day a breeze. I feel that my work makes a positive contribution to the world and I am always growing and developing in a professional capacity. I am in a deeply loving, intimate relationship. We support, nurture and respect each other, and we are always laughing and having loads of fun. We communicate clearly and we are best friends. I am close with all my family members and we are in regular contact. We are always there for one another. I am a great parent and my kids bring an abundance of joy and wonder to my life. I bring joy to my family. I have an incredible group of friends. I feel blessed that my life is so balanced and fulfilling. I have plenty of money to do whatever I want, whenever I want, and with whoever I want. I love the home I live in, and I feel safe, strong and proud of my savings, which grow every month. I take four holidays each year, both domestic and international. I love seeing new things and broadening my mind. I live a life of fun and adventure! I am always learning and growing. The more I learn, the more I want to learn. I love the person I am and I love the life I lead. I have achieved all of this, or something better.

Undertaking a process like this can seem overwhelming, and you might not know where to start, but just start! Do something! There is no right and wrong. You don't have to show anyone.

In fact, I find that once you start, you get thinking, then you get immersed, then you get creative, and then the way forward appears.

By taking the time to set 'intentions' and create a vision statement story, you help ensure you are positively influencing your own life.

Just as the five people you spend a lot of time with influence you, you also influence them and you influence yourself.

Set yourself up to live your best life and be a positive influence on others and yourself as well. It's well worth the effort.

> **Most people live — whether physically, intellectually, or morally — in a very restricted circle of their potential being. We all have reservoirs of life to draw upon of which we do not dream.**
>
> - William James

inSpired

▌Passion and Purpose

Alright, the secret of happiness is simple:
find out what you truly love to do and
then direct all of your energy towards doing it.
If you study the happiest, healthiest, most satisfied
people of our world, you will see that each and
every one of them has found their passion in life,
and then spent their days pursuing it.
This calling is almost always one that,
in some way, serves others.

- Robin Sharma

By living a life of passion and purpose, you can move from desperation to joy, from confusion to clarity, from dissatisfaction to fulfilment. By flourishing as a person, you will enrich your life. I want to encourage you to think about what you truly want in this lifetime.

Then I want to provide you with the tools and accountability to move towards that.

I believe health equals freedom.

I believe relationships equal fulfilment.

I believe a satisfying career and financial abundance create options and allow us to experience all the beauty this world has to offer.

What's the best way to lead a life of inspiration? It comes down to three things:

- Understanding your core personal values and living life directly in line with them.
- Contributing positively in the world – through your work or any other way you can share your gifts in a way that impacts others.
- Growing and evolving as a person by constantly learning, getting outside your comfort zone and setting goals in line with your values.

> **What most people don't understand is that passion is the result of action, not the cause of it.**
>
> - Mark Manson

I believe you need to determine your top values and live in line with those. Values are a lens through which we see the world and a filter through which we can make decisions.

We will always have challenges in life, but if we are living in alignment with our values, they aren't challenges at all — they are steps along the journey to fulfilment.

What's the goal here?

Is it happiness?

Happiness can be described as an 'in the moment' feeling, that is, it feels good, then passes.

I prefer to focus on something much deeper — fulfilment. Fulfilment is derived from living your life with a sense of purpose and in line with your values, while being stimulated through growth and change, rather than living a 'Groundhog Day' lifestyle.

I have invested a good deal of time and money over the years identifying my values and purpose, and identifying what lights me up and exactly why I am here on the planet.

I went through a process with an organisation called "The Brandheart Method" which helped me identify each area within the following diagram:

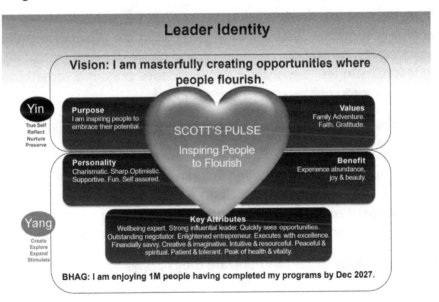

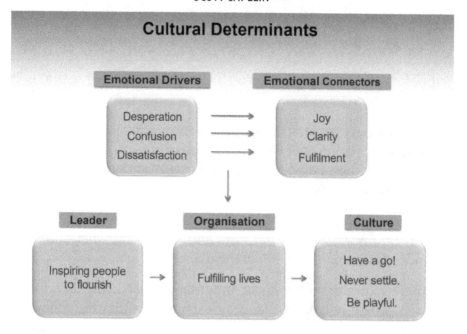

Cultural Determinants

Taking the time to refine this using the services of a professional skilled in helping someone discover their purpose in life provides a great deal of clarity, conviction, confidence, and peace of mind. One of my biggest fears in life is spending a few decades pursuing something and then finding out I was on the wrong track!

And in case you're not sure what a BHAG is, it stands for Big, Hairy, Audacious Goal!

In order to distinguish between happiness and fulfilment, I think about anyone who decides to climb Mount Everest. Imagine they are three-quarters of the way to the summit. They're cold, tired and aching after having trained for months or years to make it to the top.

During the climb, in the moment, are they happy?

Probably not!

Now imagine the satisfaction they will feel when they make it all the way to the top! Finally, imagine the sense of pride and fulfilment that stays with that person for the rest of their lives, after having achieved such a monumental challenge.

**Don't live the same year 75 times
and call it a life.**

- Robin Sharma

Think about how this achievement could change them as a person, in the most positive of ways.

Moving forward, do you think they could overcome any challenge?

Do you think they would feel a deep sense of personal pride and contentment?

Of course, they would!

Self-confidence is a function of being your best. Personal growth leads to humility because the more you learn, the more you realise you don't know — which is the opposite of being narrow-minded or having a fixed mindset.

Fulfilment is stronger than happiness. Happiness is okay, however, we can attain happiness with quick fixes.

In the early 1900's there was a famous polar explorer called Sir Ernest Shackleton. Legend has it that before embarking on one of his expeditions he placed an advertisement in The Times looking for a crew to join his ship.

The ad read:

"Men wanted for hazardous journey. Low wages, bitter cold, long hours of complete darkness. Safe return doubtful. Honour and recognition in event of success."

There were over 5,000 applicants, and from this Shackleton selected a crew of 27 people.

What kind of values did these people share?

I can only speculate; however, I dare say challenge, adventure, growth, and freedom would be among them.

There is one thing that may even outrank fulfilment — peace. Inner peace overrides everything because it means you are okay with things, regardless of how they are.

Peace quashes angst and anxiety and takes a load off your shoulders. It is the antidote to comparison and judgement and allows you to live in the present without wanting more, or wishing your days away.

My mission in life is to help people flourish. I believe the best way to be happy and fulfilled is to grow. I believe the fastest way to grow is to be pushed and held accountable for your dreams.

I believe the smartest way to get outside your comfort zone is with help from a caring, passionate mentor who has been there and done it all before. I am here to push you and support you.

I am here to hold your hand and kick your butt. I have reached a point in my life where I am equally as happy to help other people experience more abundance, joy and beauty in their lives as I am to seek more for myself. The irony is — the more people I help, the more satisfied I become.

Success, like happiness, cannot be pursued. It must ensue. And it only does so as the unintended side effect of one's personal dedication to a cause greater than oneself.

- Viktor Frankl

There was a time in my life when I had achieved what many people perceived to be 'success'. However, I felt hollow inside. I searched for solutions and ran into obstacles multiple times. It looked like I was doing well financially, but I wasn't feeling fulfilled. I wasn't feeling what I thought I'd feel as a result of my accomplishments.

I knew I was in great shape, but my relationship wasn't where I wanted it to be. I looked like I was living the high life, but I had financial issues nobody knew about, and I was being influenced by the wrong people. In short, I was out of balance. I was unaware of my core values and my purpose on this earth. I sensed I wasn't alone and I went on a mission to find clarity and experience as much joy, abundance and beauty as I could generate — for myself and for the people I loved and cared about.

I became determined to create opportunities for people and provide them with the means and the accountability to live epic lives. That is why I wrote this book.

> Money, like health, love, happiness,
> and all forms of miraculous happenings that you
> want to create for yourself, is the result of your
> living purposefully. It is not a goal unto itself.
>
> - Dr. Wayne Dyer

If you want to know where your heart
is, look where your mind goes when
it wanders.

There is a Japanese concept called *ikigai*, which loosely translates to 'a reason for being'. The word refers to having a meaningful direction or purpose in life, constituting the sense of one's life being made worthwhile and involves taking action towards achieving one's *ikigai*, resulting in satisfaction and a sense of meaning to life. (Wikipedia)

Ikigai

A JAPANESE CONCEPT MEANING "A REASON FOR BEING"

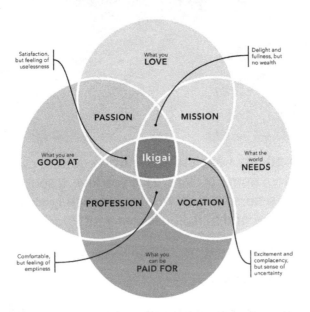

The best way to live a life of purpose is to identify your values and passions. I believe that passion, contribution and self-awareness are the keys to a beautiful life. You simply cannot go through life without identifying these critical aspects of fulfilment.

Satisfaction, fulfilment, happiness and inspiration comes from having a goal and moving towards it. Even if the attainment of the goal is a long way away. Even if you're making small progress. It's about moving towards ... moving forward. The "moving towards" is as fulfilling as the achievement of the goal. That's why we need to pursue something. Successful people attach happiness to making progress - not just the attainment of the end goal.

> **What you get will never make you happy
> in the long term. Who you become
> and what you contribute will.**
>
> - Tony Robbins

Feelings of emptiness, hopelessness and boredom, or even depression and anxiety, stem from not living a life you love. It sounds simple, but have you ever seen someone who is completely clear about what they want from life, and pursuing it voraciously, looking dejected?

There is so much juice that can be squeezed from this life.

Don't worry about failure!

Winners know there is no such thing as success and failure — only success and learning. There are not winners and losers — only winners and learners.

When you feel inspired, you love the person you are, you have a healthy respect for yourself, you only see good in the world, and you love the life you live. When someone is nasty or bitter, it's only because they are not happy within themselves. Remember: hurt people hurt people.

When you're inspired, you want to contribute positively to the world, you want to travel and have adventures and see how much you can squeeze out of life. You want to grow and develop as a person and have fun! You see someone who has purchased a great car or a beautiful home and you are really happy for them! There's a saying that many people "tiptoe through life to arrive safely at death".

And there's a Japanese proverb that says: "Only staying active will make you want to live a hundred years". Japanese people believe that if you stop being active, your level of purpose in the world will be reduced, which is a catalyst for mental and physical decline.

I promise you won't regret aspiring to all of this. I'm part realist, part idealist and entirely passionate about making things happen. Too many people are not living fulfilling lives and it's just not good enough. If you want to open your eyes and learn a whole lot about yourself, take the first steps towards designing your dream life.

Who is the most important person in the organization? Everyone.

In his book, Teaching the Elephant to Dance, author Jim Belasco tells the story of Dr. Denton Cooley, the famous heart surgeon.

One day Belasco noticed Dr Cooley having a conversation with the hospital janitor that lasted around five minutes. Belasco was curious and after they finished speaking he went over to the cleaner and said "That was a long conversation"

The man replied, "Yes, Dr. Cooley and I talk quite often."

Then Belasco asked, "What exactly do you do at the hospital?'

The man replied, "We save lives."

In the best organizations, there is no such thing as them and us; there is only "we" - all of us working together.

In the big picture everyone has a piece to the puzzle...Everyone, including and perhaps especially you, makes a difference.

I love this story. The cleaner at the hospital had the same sense of ownership and pride in what he did as the doctors, nurses and other hospital staff.

The man in the story doesn't simply think of himself as a cleaner, but as a vital member of the team, with purpose!

> Whatever you feel compelled to do, be it writing music, designing software, doing floral arrangements, cleaning teeth, or driving a taxi - do it with your unique flair. Being creative means trusting your inner calling, ignoring criticism or judgment, and releasing resistance to your natural talents.
>
> - Dr. Wayne Dyer

What is the first step?

The choice is yours. You could do any one of a number of things, including:

- working through the goal-setting (intention-setting) exercises in the previous chapter
- following the steps in the previous chapter to create a vision for your life
- booking a call with me
- doing the Dream Life Design program (inlifecoaching.com.au)
- identifying your 'Top 6' personal core values and analysing whether the way you spend your time reflects those values
- asking yourself how you could spend more time living in line with the values you listed in the point above

I do this work because I love it. I wake up excited every day. I want the same for you.

There's a classic book, Kon-Tiki, where the lead character sails a balsawood raft on a 4,000-mile journey from South America to the Polynesian Islands. All sorts of factors occurred that he could not have anticipated – the wood expanded, tightening the raft and making it stronger; flying fish landed on the raft every day – assisting him on his journey. These are examples of how the way forward can appear.

Following your heart, and contributing to causes greater than yourself is the key to fulfilment and contentment.

> **Whatever you feel within you as your calling - whatever makes you feel alive - know in your heart that this excitement is all the evidence you need to have your inner passion become reality. This is precisely how creation works...and it's that energy that harmonizes with the way. The right way.**
>
> - Tao Te Ching

The Courage to Change and Have a Go!

> My father could have been a great comedian,
> but he didn't believe that was possible
> for him, and so he made a conservative choice.
> Instead, he got a safe job as an accountant.
> When I was 12 years old, he was let go from that
> safe job, and our family had to do whatever we
> could to survive. I learned many great lessons
> from my father, not the least of which was that you
> can fail at what you don't want, so you might as
> well take a chance on doing what you love.
>
> - Jim Carrey

...biggest topics in my work is change. As a Health and
...hen I meet a new client, it is when they have made
...tion – their first step being to work with me as
...nd grow.

...the first big step, enlisting me to work
...t should be acknowledged, because it is
...ry move.

If you're brave enough to say "goodbye",
life will reward you with a new "hello".

- Paulo Coelho

Change happens when the pain
of staying the same is greater
than the pain of change.

- Tony Robbins

It is secure and comfortable staying where you are, even when
ot 100% happy. Change is hard, and whilst you may wan
itive progress in your life, you might not be sure how

Things are never happy at
the moment of change.
But sometimes that unhappiness
just means that you're doing
something worth doing.

A Baseball Analogy

I used to play and coach a lot of baseball. I played at a high level in my younger years. In my health and life coaching role, seeing people strive for a richer life, I have often felt that people see themselves as the batter looking to hit a home run in a game of baseball.

They say things like, "If I could just get that new job", or "It will all fall into place when I meet the right person", and "I'll be happy when I lose the weight".

People tend to look for that one big thing they think will make them feel better. Yet it's the focus on the limitations of where they currently are that creates spiritual resistance and repels the manifestation of what they want.

Is that a little heavy? Let me try and explain.

You cannot push towards what you want if you are focused on the negatives associated with what you don't want and where you currently are. It's called resistance. It's the number one reason people do not achieve the goals they set for themselves. Resistance is subtle and comes in many forms.

Perhaps you want to be wealthy but are critical or jealous of the person you see driving a Ferrari.

Can you see what's happening here?

You may want to attract wealth but you are associating negative energy with the attainment of wealth. You might want to be skinny but mock a slim person. Or you may want to travel the world or run a marathon but, either consciously or subconsciously, you do not believe you can do it.

It's all resistance, and it's the ultimate manifestation blocker. What do I mean by manifestation? It's when you bring your desires to reality or fruition.

There are many more forces at work than we can see and, as mere mortals, we do not have all the information. Has something ever happened to you that you didn't want, but two years later you find yourself in an amazing place you would not have been in, if that 'bad event' had not occurred?

Maybe you lost your job, only to find a better one?

Maybe you were dumped by the person you loved, even though it wasn't the greatest relationship, then you met the partner of your dreams?

Back to the baseball analogy! **You aren't batting in the baseball game, you are pitching!** All you need to do is keep throwing pitches. The Universe is batting, and it will decide which ball to hit for the home run. Keep trying, with an open mind, and don't get too attached to outcomes.

There is no possibility of a home run without the pitches. Rather than setting goals – set intentions. Do your best to be free of all forms of resistance, and enjoy watching everything unfold.

Check out this story which illustrates why we should not be elated with the highs in life or depressed with the lows.

"An old farmer had worked his crops for many years. One day his horse ran away. Upon hearing the news, his neighbors came to visit.
"Such bad luck", they said sympathetically.

"Maybe", the farmer replied. The next morning the horse returned, bringing with it three other wild horses. "How wonderfull!" his neighbors exclaimed.

"Maybe", replied the old man. The following day, his son tried to ride one of the untamed horses, was thrown, and broke his leg. The neighbors again came to offer sympathies on his misfortune.

"Maybe", answered the farmer. The day after, military officers came to the village to draft young men into the army. Seeing that the son's leg was broken, they passed him by. The neighbors congratulated the farmer on how well things had turned out. "Maybe", said the farmer".

Sometimes, I ask people a very general question to gauge where they are at with their overall levels of life satisfaction and fulfilment. The question is: On a scale of one to ten, how happy are you right now with your life?

There are all sorts of answers, ranging from two to nine. For some reason, very few people think a ten is possible. Most commonly, the response is six or seven but the problem with sixes and sevens is you're not a four or five out of ten (which is good), but you're not an eight, nine, or ten either, and at six and seven things aren't bad enough to make you want to instigate action to improve.

When you're at the lower end, it's like, "I'll do whatever it takes!" People can languish in the middle zone for years, doing nothing. Wouldn't you rather shoot for the stars, have fun doing it, stuff up a few things along the way, learn a lot, and grow as a person?

> **Most men lead lives
> of quiet desperation...
> and go to the grave with
> the song still in them.**
>
> - Henry David Threau

Ask yourself now, what score you would rate your life happiness, on a scale from 1 to 10. It's a general question, so a ballpark answer is fine.

How do you feel about your response?

Now answer these questions:

- Do you feel you have more in you?
- Do you feel trapped in your job?
- Are you happy with your body?
- Are you being the best parent you can be?
- Do you have holidays booked that you can look forward to?
- Are you happy in your relationship?

I heard a story recently about a 60-year-old woman who divorced her husband. The man had not been kind to her for most of her life. One of her friends commented, "Why would you separate now? Who is going to look after you when you're old?"

What if I fail?

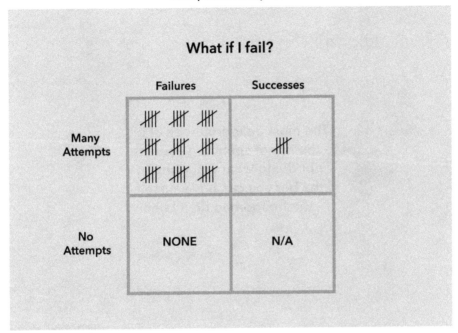

	Failures	Successes
Many Attempts	╫╫ ╫╫ ╫╫ ╫╫ ╫╫ ╫╫ ╫╫ ╫╫ ╫╫	╫╫
No Attempts	NONE	N/A

This comment implies that staying in an unhappy marriage is better than being on your own, or that you should stay with someone for the sake of convenience. The man had never looked after this woman during their entire relationship, so it was doubtful he would begin once they reached their twilight years.

Our heart knows what we want. On a spiritual level, we have an 'inner being' or a 'higher self'. When we experience negative emotion it's our higher self letting us know we are out of alignment with what we truly want. We often use logic to talk ourselves out of following our heart.

The idea is to identify what would make you happy and pursue it with a smart approach. There is a great deal of fear associated with the unknown, but abundance, joy and beauty are found on the other side of the unknown.

Don't do nothing and expect things to get better. Don't resign yourself to where you are and don't settle for less. There are 168 hours in a week. You might work 40 of them. If you're lucky, you sleep for 56 hours. That leaves 72 remaining hours.

**The most dangerous risk of all
- the risk of spending your life
not doing what you want on
the bet you can buy yourself
the freedom to do it later.**

Of those, you should dedicate five to exercise.

Can you dedicate ten hours a week to getting your side hustle off the ground?

Or is it better to spend those ten hours watching Netflix?

This is oversimplifying it, and it's a little bit cheeky. If you're a single mum working full-time, there might not be much spare time at all. The point is – we make time for whatever we feel is most important.

Can you fit your exercise in?

There's never a perfect time to make all this happen. When is 'now' the perfect time?

If you're a busy person, there is never a perfect time to exercise. You might think you can't do it because you have to get lots of other things in. Just get your exercise in and watch how you magically get those other things done anyway.

"Live life fully while you're here. Experience everything. Take care of yourself and your friends. Have fun, be crazy, be weird. Go out and screw up! You're going to anyway, so you might as well enjoy the process. Take the opportunity to learn from your mistakes: find the cause of your problem and eliminate it. Don't try to be perfect; just be an excellent example of being human."

-Tony Robbins

Limiting Beliefs

Many of us have limiting beliefs. A limiting belief is a thought or opinion that you think is true, however, it may not necessarily be the case.

You might say "I couldn't take six months off work", or "I will never get a better job than the one I have, so I should just stay here". Limiting beliefs prevent you from moving forward in life.

Over the years I have helped countless people achieve their weight loss goals, and at that point, we set other objectives. A common endeavour has always been to enter and complete a half-marathon. Running 21.1km is a huge achievement, however, the most common initial reaction is "I couldn't possibly run that far", with a few expletives thrown in.

My standard reply is "Well, you won't run that far with that attitude". So, we train for it, and everyone completes it, and I ask them to never again tell me that they cannot do something. What limiting beliefs might you have that are keeping you stuck?

Belief and Faith

A lack of belief can like a ball and chain holding you back. It could be a lack of belief in yourself, or a lack of belief that a better way or better outcome is possible.

If you're into The Bible, you can see evidence of the importance of belief. In the book of Mark (9:23) Jesus says "If you can believe, all things are possible to him who believes".

On other occasions, Jesus also said "As ye believe, so shall it be done unto you".

There's a passage from the book of Hebrews (11:1) which I love that says "Faith is the assurance of things hoped for, the conviction of things not seen", meaning that whilst you cannot see what you desire, you must believe it will come to fruition. You've probably heard people say "I'll believe it when I see it", however ironically the reverse is true.

To see it, you must first believe it. Everything happens twice - first in your mind, then in reality. Whatever you want in life must happen in your mind first, so start imagining, visualising, and daydreaming.

American minister Norman Vincent Peale is quoted as saying "This is one of the greatest laws of the universe: Briefly and simply stated it says that if you think in negative terms, you will get negative results. If you think in positive terms, you will achieve positive results".

The following images depict our thoughts shooting out into the universe, which will in turn bring back to us what we are focusing on, be it good or bad.

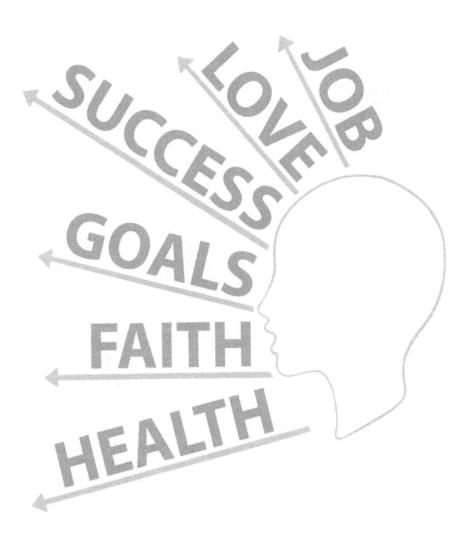

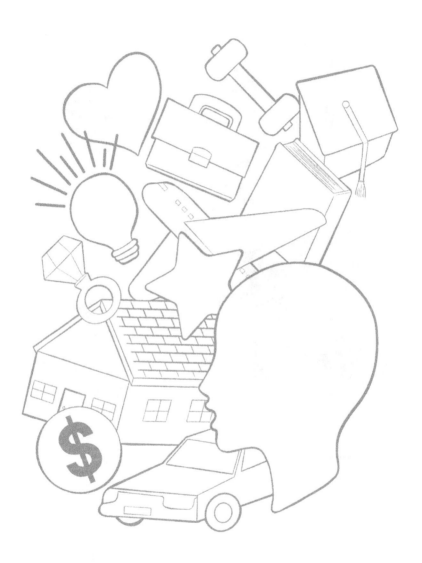

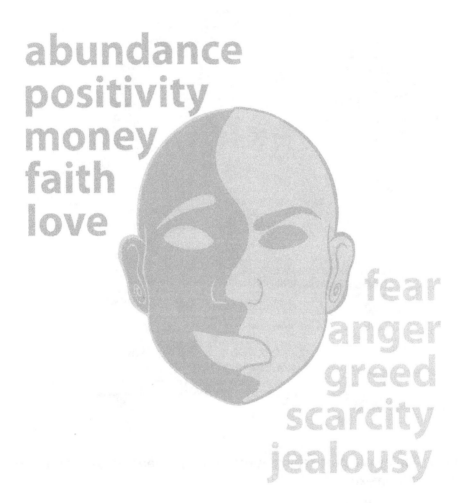

abundance
positivity
money
faith
love

fear
anger
greed
scarcity
jealousy

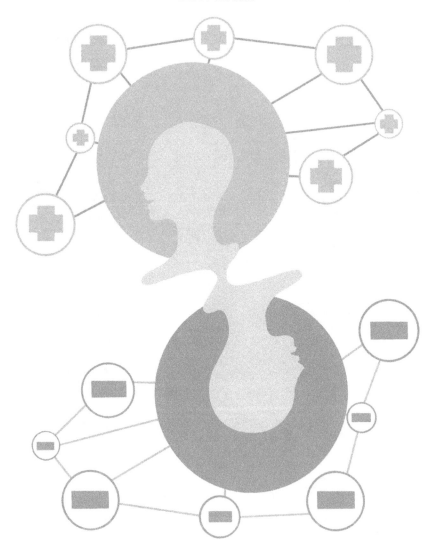

Mike Dooley is a best-selling author, entrepreneur, speaker, and Law of Attraction expert.

He says "Thoughts become things, so choose the good ones!"

Shakespeare said, "our doubts are traitors and make us lose the good we oft might win by fearing to attempt".

It makes sense that the first step towards a more abundant life is the unwavering belief that it can happen.

These topics are touched on in a little more detail in the next chapter on Mindset.

> The secret to happiness is freedom...
> And the secret to freedom is courage.
>
> - Thucydides

Winners Find Solutions

Find the answers! Instead of saying "I can't do it", ask yourself "How can I do it?"

Our brain is wired to find solutions.

Ask it questions!

Don't have a pain in your shoulder for four years and live with it. See a Chinese medicine doctor. Or a naturopath.

Make it your mission to have a fully functioning, pain-free body. Strive to be more flexible, mobile and energetic, and live with a higher degree of vitality. Travel, take up a new hobby, open an online business, and if it doesn't work, fail quietly and quickly, and move on.

People say, "I've tried everything". So, I ask what they've tried. As it turns out, they've often only tried two things. If your knees or back are bad, go to every length to fix them.

Have you tried a sugar-free diet?

Consider a knee replacement.

See a movement coach.

Try Pilates and yoga.

A chiro.

See a physiotherapist or osteopath.

If you don't try everything, refer back to your values and you'll realise peak health isn't one of them. You'll always be in pain or without the flexibility to put your shoes on. Raise your standards. Find the answers!

> **Wisdom is looking back at your life and realising that every single event, person, place and idea was part of the perfected experience you needed to build your dream. Not one was a mistake.**
>
> - John Demartini

On a broader level, look to enrich your life with goals, and travel, and associate with new people who encourage you and make you want to become better.

Speaking to family and friends isn't always the answer. When I talk to my friends, they say, "Relax man, you're killing it!" I like to talk to someone external to my immediate circle – someone who is objective and unattached to my results.

Someone skilled in asking the right questions so I can come up with the answers myself. Associate with people who make you lift your game. Hang out with people who earn in a day what you earn in a month. If you want to run fast, run with faster runners!

PERSONAL GROWTH AND FULFILMENT MODEL

COMFORT ZONE	THE UNKNOWN	HAPPINESS
		EXCITEMENT
		PRIDE
		ABUNDANCE
BOREDOM	FEAR	JOY
APATHY		FULFILMENT
MEDIOCRITY		SATISFACTION

I come across some people who are stuck in a rut with their health and their life overall, and it only seems to be getting deeper. Many of us could do with a complete lifestyle change.

Could you change jobs?

Live a simpler life and move to the country or a quieter town on the coast?

Could you buy a cheaper car and alleviate financial stress?

More exercise, dieting, getting a promotion at work and buying a bigger house can often be just more things that are adding to your headspace and stress load.

It's not always practical to leave a job if you need the money. The good news is you will probably be alive for another 40 years and you can plan another path to pursue.

Can you spend the next 12 months setting yourself up for a change?

Can you develop another skill?

There's an inspiring book called The Million-Dollar One-Person Business by Elaine Pofeldt which highlights the proliferation of people starting their own business and generating over $1,000,000 per year in revenue.

The book tag line is "Make great money. Work the way you like. Have the life you want". There are worse things you could do than read this book.

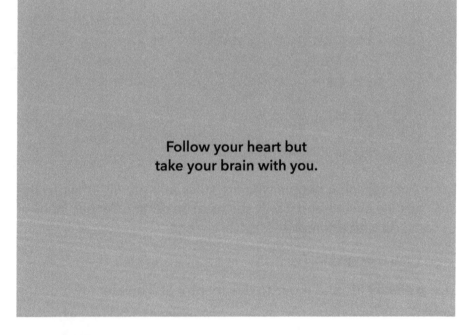

Follow your heart but take your brain with you.

Joseph Campbell gave the message more eloquently when he said, "Follow your bliss". He was an American professor who dedicated his life to studying the human experience

> If you do follow your bliss you put yourself on
> a kind of track that has been there all the while,
> waiting for you, and the life that you ought to be
> living is the one you are living. When you can
> see that, you begin to meet people who are
> in the field of your bliss, and they open the doors
> to you. I say, follow your bliss and don't be afraid,
> and doors will open where you didn't
> know they were going to be.
>
> - Joseph Campbell

Campbell stated there are spiritual and serendipitous reasons for following your bliss. He said when you pursue what you love, you will come across the people, ideas, time, money, resources and whatever else you need to bring your dreams to fruition.

I love the way he says that doors will open where previously there were no doors.

Pretty cool, hey?

It's almost like we are rewarded by the universe for having the courage to step outside our comfort zone and pursue our passion.

Wouldn't you rather regret the things you did, than the things you didn't do?

Steve Jobs was also a believer in not following the norms of society. He said that we all have the power to achieve wonderful things, and we shouldn't limit ourselves.

If we are all going to be dead in 50 years, doesn't it make sense to try as much as we can when we are alive?

> # When you want something, all the universe conspires in helping you to achieve it.
>
> -Paulo Coelho, The Alchemist

Napoleon Hill said, "Whatever the mind can conceive and believe, it can achieve". There are a few elements to that quote, and the part most people find challenging is believing they can do something that may seem scary.

The universe has thousands of ways of bringing desires to reality, and our main task is to identify what we want, believe it's possible and then take a little action to create some momentum.

When you grow up you tend to get told that the world is the way it is and your life is just to live your life inside the world. Try not to bash into the walls too much. Try to have a nice family life, have fun, save a little money. That's a very limited life. Life can be much broader once you discover one simple fact: Everything around you that you call life was made up by people that were no smarter than you. And you can change it, you can influence it... Once you learn that, you'll never be the same again.

-Steve Jobs

I love this poem:

"I bargained with Life for a penny,
And Life would pay no more,
However I begged at evening
When I counted my scanty store;

For Life is just an employer,
He gives you what you ask,
But once you have set the wages,
Why, you must bear the task.

I worked for a menial's hire,
Only to learn, dismayed,
That any wage I had asked of Life,
Life would have paid."

-Jessie B. Rittenhouse

So, let's set our sights on something big! Let's raise our level of expectation around what we can get from this life! It really does provide us with a great deal of drive, passion and inspiration.

Big intentions result in personal growth, which builds wisdom, confidence and character. Even failures are only learning lessons, so we really don't have anything to lose ... only great things to gain!

Get to the end of your life and be able to say that you did everything you could with every gift you had!

> **You get what you expect, have you noticed that?**
> **You expect to survive, and so you do. You expect**
> **to have a roof over your head, and so you do.**
> **You expect to live alright, and so you do.**
> **But you don't expect extraordinary things, so they**
> **don't come. You don't expect magnificent money**
> **to flow into your experience and so it**
> **cannot get in. The only thing that comes to you**
> **is what you are expecting to come to you.**
>
> - Abraham Hicks

If I had to sum up the theme of my coaching work over the years in one word, it would be 'change'. People enquire about using the services of a coach when they are wanting to change. It always surprises me how we are not prepared for big changes, even when we can see them coming.

We can see the weight increasing, we can see the relationship has lost its spark, we know the kids will leave home, we know we don't love our job or it might not be secure. I see the effects that levels of uncertainty have on people in the areas of health, relationships and careers.

Change is scary. It is natural to want to avoid it. There's a reason the 'comfort zone' has its name – it's comfortable! And comfortable is nice – it's just not fulfilling.

> There is no passion to be found
> playing small - in settling for
> a life that is less than the one
> you are capable of living.
>
> - Nelson Mandela

I often feel there are two types of mental strength:

1. Being strong when you have no choice, such as a death in the family, or your partner walking out on you or having to support your family.

2. Being strong when you do have a choice, but you've chosen to stay in the easy option. This is what requires real strength of character, and this is where people can be stuck for years. This is where many people DO NOT show mental strength, because they DO stay in the unhappy yet familiar place. It is in these situations that real mental strength is required.

If you've had a recurring thought over a long period of time, it's probably right and it's time to act. On the flip side, if you've had a goal for a long time and you've made no progress, you either need accountability or some kind of help to get you to take action.

Or – it's not that important to you, so do yourself a favour and forget about it.

A recurring thought is a message from the universe trying to awaken you to a new possibility. Think of it as the universe giving you a tap on the shoulder.

If you don't take notice of the tap, you eventually get hit with a baseball bat. If the baseball bat doesn't wake you up, sooner or later you get hit by a Mack truck.

Don't wait until you get hit by a truck (metaphorically speaking) to make a change.

> It's the possibility of having a dream come true that makes life interesting.
>
> -Paulo Coelho, The Alchemist

People can't pinpoint why they make bad food decisions or poor life decisions. They are bored. Uninspired. Low in confidence. Lacking purpose. Whatever the reason, food is comfort and connection.

That's not all of it, but it's part of it. Even worse – are you a 'passenger' in your own journey?

Are you in control of your life or at the mercy of whatever happens to you on a daily basis?

There's never a perfect time to make a positive change – and nobody is going to do it for you.

Are you living your dreams or just helping someone else achieve theirs?

In fifty years, we won't be around, and nobody will really care that much anyway. So – have a crack now.

The opposite for courage is not cowardice, it is conformity. Even a dead fish can go with the flow.

- Jim Hightower

Fast forward to the last day of your life...

...What will have been most important? Then make that important now.

-Robin Sharma

Mindset Mastery

A beautiful day begins with a beautiful mindset. When you wake up, take a second to think about what a privilege it is to simply be alive & healthy. The moment we start acting like life is a blessing I assure you it will start to feel like one.

> # If you only say one prayer in a day, make it thank you.
>
> -Rumi

What Does 'Mindset' Mean?

Simply put, mindset is a way of thinking that shapes the way you look at the world and the events that happen. Your mindset is your collection of beliefs that colour your thought habits. Your thought habits affect how you think, how you feel, and what you do.

Your mindset impacts how you make sense of the world and how you make sense of yourself.

So it makes sense to ask yourself "What kind of mindset would I like to have?"

What qualities and characteristics would I like to embody in order to help me get through life in a way that makes me feel strong and confident?

What will get me through the ups and downs I will inevitably experience?"

I like to break a healthy mindset down into the following seven parts, with each part having three sub-parts.

232

1. Values, Vision and Vitality

Understand your values and live in line with them. Have a clear vision for your future and know exactly what kind of life you want to lead.

When creating your life vision don't get too caught up in the details or how you're going to make it happen - the detail and worrying about the "how" can be a dream killer, and those details can wait for later. Be in the best shape you can be and have enormous levels of energy and vitality.

Dr Martin Luther King is one of the most famous and influential men in history. He had a vision, backed by conviction, faith, and belief.

He said, "I have a dream!" He never said he had a plan! He stood up for his values and inspired millions of people.

> Values are like fingerprints.
> Nobodies are the same, but you leave
> them all over everything you do.
>
> - Elvis Presley

2. Goals, Gratitude and Growth

Have a clear set of goals that will inspire you. Be grateful and appreciate every little good thing in your life, regardless of the overall position you are in. Always be growing and developing as a person.

Are the happiest people the most grateful, or are the most grateful people the happiest?

Definitely the latter!

When you train your mind to look for the gifts in every situation – both good and bad – it will transcend your life to a higher dimension.

**If you are not growing,
you are dying.**

- Tony Robbins.

Gratitude is the best medicine. It heals your mind, your body and your spirit. And attracts more things to be grateful for.

3. Passion, Positivity and Purpose

Live a life of passion, doing the things you love. Be positive! Fill your mind with inspiring things and avoid negativity at all costs.

Live with a sense of purpose that comes from doing things that make this world a better place.

There's a school of thought that says: to live the life you want and manifest the things you desire, you have to feel good as much as you can.

Can it be as simple as that?

From a 'law of attraction' perspective, you cannot attract something good while feeling something bad, so do things that make you feel good!

The fastest way to get to where you want to be
is to focus positively about where you are.

- Abraham Hicks

To live life to the fullest, you must stand guard
at the gate of your garden and let only the very
best information enter. You truly cannot afford
the luxury of a negative thought – not even one.
The most joyful, dynamic, and contented people
of this world are no different from you
or me in terms of their makeup.

- From The Monk Who Sold His Ferrari

4. Connection, Contribution and Confidence

Connect to the things you love. Connect with your partner. Spend your life doing things you feel congruent with. Give – contribution is one of your highest innate needs and it explodes your feelings of self-worth.

When you live a life you love and do things that fill you with happiness and pride, you will exude an aura of confidence, and that's sexy!

> **Your level of happiness, fulfilment, and whatever success means to you is directly proportionate to your level of personal growth and the value you add to the world.**
>
> - Scott Capelin

5. Strength, Self-Image and Surrender

You have to be mentally strong. Accept what is. Have the attitude that you can endure anything. Love the person you are. It's hard for anyone else to love you if you can't lead the way.

Relax and know that some things will go your way and some won't, but everything is going to be alright. Life is full of ups and downs and that won't change, so it's not about whether you are up or down, it's about how you react to the setbacks. It's okay to get upset or disappointed – it's normal – just don't stay there for long.

Have a mind that is open to everything
and attached to nothing.

- Dr. Wayne Dyer

6. Focus, Faith and Fulfilment

Gain clarity regarding who you are and where you want to go. Believe it is all possible. The ultimate goal is to be fulfilled and that is even more important than being happy.

Take the first step in faith.
You don't have to see the whole staircase,
just take the first step.

- Martin Luther King

7. Affirmations, Abundance and Action

Repeat positive thoughts to yourself so they embed into your subconscious mind. Believe that there is so much out there for you and everyone else. You really can be, do and have whatever you want from this life. Take action. Nothing happens by itself and nobody else will do it for you.

In summary, when you think about mindset, think about the way you want to look at the world, how you react to the things that happen in your life and the way you feel about yourself. It helps all areas of life if your mindset is strong, positive and optimistic.

If you have a strong sense of self-belief that is mixed with hope and faith, and if you feel like the universe is a friendly place and all the help you need is available to you, then you can achieve anything you put your mind to.

That's the kind of mindset we must aspire to. These topics are expanded upon in much greater detail in my book, *Fit to Flourish: 7 Simple Steps to Mindset Mastery*.

There are so many beautiful reasons to be happy.

Carol Dweck on Mindset

Professor Carol Dweck, an American psychologist and author of "Mindset", found that we all have different beliefs about the underlying nature of ability.

She established that people with a "growth mindset" believe that intelligence and abilities can be developed through effort, persistence, trying different strategies and learning from mistakes.

On the other hand, people with a "fixed mindset" believe that intelligence and abilities are fixed traits; something that you are born with and that you can't really do anything about.

Clearly, a growth mindset is more conducive to progress and success in any endeavour.

> Quality questions create a quality life.
> Successful people ask better questions,
> and as a result, they get better answers.
>
> - Anthony Robbins

A quick note about goals, success, and belief

The best definition of success I have come across came from one of the fathers of personal development, Earl Nightingale, who said that "Success is the progressive realisation of a worthy goal or ideal".

He also uses the analogy of a ship sailing off into the sea, and says that if you have a goal and a plan it's like the ship having a captain and a crew, which means it will stay on course and reach its destination.

What do you think will happen to that ship if there was no captain or crew?

It will sail off to nowhere in particular, and probably crash or sink, or at the very least wander aimlessly and waste a lot of time. That's what life is like without goals. This information comes from Earl Nightingales book called The Strangest Secret.

You can find the audio for free on YouTube. It's only 30 minutes long and filled with eye-opening, practical tips you can implement immediately.

Earl goes on to describe a survey asking people why they get up in the morning and go to work or do whatever it is that you do.

He says that 95% of people had no idea, and many people said "Because everyone else does". He says that whether you are an accountant, a mother, coach, salesperson or plumber, aim to be the best one you can be. And importantly, make sure that whatever you do is something that you have chosen because you are passionate about it.

> Attitude is a choice.
> Happiness is a choice.
> Optimism is a choice.
> Kindness is a choice.
> Giving is a choice.
> Respect is a choice.
> Whatever choice you make makes you.
> Choose wisely.
>
> - Roy T. Bennett

The biggest key to achieving a strong mindset is to flick away every negative thought and replace it with gratitude.

Do this over, and over, and over, until it becomes second nature and your default mode is gratitude and appreciation. You can't be angry and grateful at the same time.

You can't be fearful and appreciative at the same time. You can't be jealous and grateful at the same time. Gratitude is the antidote to all the yucky emotions.

You get more of what you are grateful for. The more you practice gratitude the more attuned you will become to negative thoughts of yourself and others.

Most people don't even realise they are being negative and when you mention it to them, it is almost a surprise. Think of your mind like a fertile garden and don't let any weeds in there. You want to be a person that other people want to be around.

There is a gift in every negative situation, you just need to take a moment to look for it.

Start a gratitude diary and write down five things you are grateful for every night before you go to sleep. When you wake up in the morning let your first thought be "thank you", and think of 5 things that you appreciate in your life, starting with your warm, comfortable bed!

Gratitude is the healthiest of all human emotions.

The more you express gratitude for what you have, the more likely you will have even more to express gratitude for.

-Zig Ziglar

Every time you praise something, every time you appreciate something, every time you feel good about something, you are telling the Universe, "More of this, please."

-Abraham Hicks

If you have a broken mindset,
you really only have two choices.
You can learn how to overcome it, improving
your life or you can keep it, and limit yourself
from achieving your life goals.

- Brandon Carter

Your mind is a garden
Your thoughts are the seeds
You can grow flowers
Or
You can grow weeds.

- Ritu Ghatourey

We vibrate energy, and the energy we give out comes back to us. The following diagram shows the frequencies at which we can vibrate. Where do you see yourself on this scale?

Emotion:		Frequency:
Enlightenment	o	700+
Peace	o	600
Joy	o	540
Love	o	500
Reason	o	400
Acceptance	o	350
Willingness	o	310
Neutrality	o	250
Courage	o	200
Pride	o	175
Anger	o	150
Desire	o	125
Fear	o	100
Grief	o	75
Apathy	o	50
Guilt	o	30
Shame	o	20

Expanded

Contracted

Virtual Scale of Consciousness

(E)motions = Energy in Motion. Energy Vibrates at a certain Frequency. The Law of Vibration activates the Law of Attraction & through the Law of Deservedness you attract what you send out by the Emotions you hold in your body.

(Diagram of the Hawkins Scale of Consciousness)

Miserable people want you to lower your vibration to meet their own. This will make them like you more, but it's also a foolproof way to block your own personal growth. You need to train the people around you to meet you at your level. Be compassionate about where they are in their journey, but you must stay strong and never lower your vibration. If they are drowning, it won't serve you to jump in the pool and drown with them.

Most people do not realize that
as they continue to find things to
complain about, they disallow
their own physical well-being.
Many do not realize that before
they were complaining about an
aching body or a chronic disease,
they were complaining about
many other things first. It does
not matter if the object of your
complaint is about someone you
are angry with, behavior in others
that you believe is wrong, or
something wrong with your own
physical body. Complaining is
complaining, and it disallows
improvement.

-Abraham Hicks

Viktor Frankl's classic book, *Man's Search for Meaning*, states, "The greatest power we possess is the power to choose". Frankl was an Austrian psychologist and a Holocaust survivor. He developed the belief that whilst everything may be taken away from us, the one thing that cannot be taken is our attitude.

He also says that your level of personal motivation, fulfilment, clarity and drive comes from knowing your life's purpose in the first place, and living a life that is meaningful to you.

We can choose good health, we can choose better decisions, we can choose a better life, and when we make those decisions, unseen forces gather to bring our desires to fruition.

Examples of switching a negative to a positive include:

- Saying, "I'm squeezing a lot into life," instead of "I'm tired"
- Thinking about how fortunate you are to have a warm bed, a roof over your head and running hot water ready to go, instead of focusing on how early it is and how comfortable you are when you wake up and don't want to get out of bed
- Being grateful that you can exercise, instead of saying, "I don't feel like exercising".
- Being grateful that you have two arms, two legs and eyes that can see, instead of being unhappy with your body
- Reminding yourself how blessed you are to be a parent, rather than complaining about your kids
- Appreciating the fact you are employed and have a regular income, rather than saying, "I don't want to go to work"

Attitude is everything. And your mood is a choice.

With everything that has
happened to you, you can either
feel sorry for yourself, or treat
what has happened as a gift.
Everything is either an opportunity
to grow, or an obstacle
to keep you from growing.
You get to choose.

- Wayne Dyer

I don't have any problems. I have a few
challenges though. I don't like problems,
but I love a challenge!

- Scott Capelin

Acknowledging the good that you
already have in your life is the
foundation for all abundance.

-Eckhart Tolle

Curating Your Dream Life by Planning Perfect Days

Daily and Annual Calendar Planning

Recently, I asked a friend, "How was your day yesterday?"

I actually asked him to give it a score on a scale of one to ten. He replied with seven.

I asked him, "What would have made it a nine?"

He said, "It would have been a nine if I'd gone for a walk with my headphones on early in the morning, called my father to say hello, spent half an hour with my young kids, and even had a massage."

I asked him if he could have planned all this in, and he said yes.

This brings us to the topic of this chapter — planning your perfect days to curate the dream life you most desire.

There are activities we can do daily, weekly, monthly and annually that can make our life so much richer. Right now, I would like you to make a list of things you can insert into your day, week, month or year, in order to increase the amount of joy in your life.

> Imagine you're on your death bed & standing around your death bed are the ghosts representing your unfulfilled potential, the ghosts of the ideas & dreams you never acted on, the ghosts of the talents & gifts you didn't use. They are standing around your bed angry, disappointed, and upset.
> They say, "We came to you because you could have brought us to life & now we have to go to the grave together."
> Today I ask you, how many ghosts are going to be around your bed when your time comes?
>
> - Les Brown

Two of my clients are a married couple who, more often than not, seem uninspired by life. Recently, I asked them what they had planned for the year ahead, and whether they had any holidays booked.

I asked them what they were looking forward to. "Nothing much," they said, with sloth-like enthusiasm.

Wow! No wonder they aren't excited about life! I asked, "Why not?"

They said that between work and their child, it all seems too hard to organise.

As it turns out, a lot of things are hard for them, like exercising, eating healthily and remaining positive.

With another client, part of our process was to write down five things he was grateful for each day.

"Five!" he exclaimed.

"Every day?

How can I come up with that many things?"

Well, it's not that hard, and you can repeat the same thing often. You have ears that can hear and fingers that move. You have a roof over your head, money in the bank, and there's probably a few people who care about you.

We live in a country that is safe and free, where the weather is great and there's an abundance of opportunity. This guy had a car, healthy kids, a lovely partner and loads of support.

We don't have to look far to find the good stuff. Perhaps it's our primal brain, hardwired for survival, that makes us look for danger and negatives first, or maybe it's the news telling us there's a crisis coming, or the people we associate with that like talking about their problems ... whatever it is, focusing on what's missing only brings us more of what's missing.

You cannot get to abundance from lack. You cannot attract happiness while having thoughts of unhappiness. When that's the case, you're out of alignment and you are defeated before you've begun. I'm talking about everything here: relationships, life goals, health, weight, money, your dream job ...

I don't believe in living every day like it's your last. If that were the case, I would suggest you put this book down right now! However, I do like to think about living every year like it's your last. I encourage you to fast-forward in your mind to your last days on this earth and ask yourself what is most important to you. Then, make it important now.

Here's a little list to get you thinking.

Daily Activities

- Exercise
- Coffee at a café
- Phone call with a friend
- Cuddling your kids

Weekly Activities

- Massage
- Date night
- Restaurant dinner
- Yoga class

Monthly Activities

- Weekend away
- Dinner with friends
- Have family over for a barbecue
- Go see a movie

Annual Activities

- Overseas holiday
- New car
- Skydiving

We can do anything if we put our minds to it.
Take your old life, then you put a line through it.

- Benny Blanco, Halsey, and Khalid

The things that are easy to do, such as booking a massage or organising a dinner date, are also easy not to do. I was speaking to a client, Sophie, recently about keeping the flame alive in your intimate relationship.

She is 51 years old and was divorced 12 years ago. She said she has a lot of divorced friends and they have started new relationships and are commenting on how new and fresh everything feels.

She also said that, in her experience, the reason her previous relationship became old and stale is that she and her partner never did anything that was new and fresh!

I do a lot of work with married couples in their 30's and 40's with kids, and also a lot of work with people in their 50's and 60's whose kids are now adults. I have a financial planner called Chris, who is almost 70 years old. He calls the years with young kids, the 'beautiful chaos'.

In those time-poor years, we are trying to raise a young family, build some wealth and take care of our health. I use the analogy of juggling the three balls (family, fitness and finances) – inevitably, we are dropping one or more of those balls. We can't drop the kids because they rely on us.

We can't leave our jobs because we need the money. It's in these years that health and wellness can fall by the wayside, and it's also when couples can grow distant.

I have experienced that myself. With desire and planning, we can fit in everything that is important to us and live a rich and fulfilling life.

Imagine seeing your entire year mapped out with big holidays, small weekends away and a daily structure that you love and that doesn't make you yearn for the weekend. It can all be done, but nobody is going to plan your dream life except you!

> My goal is to be filthy rich. Rich in adventure, in health, in knowledge, in laughter, in family and in love.

Dream Boards

A dream board, or vision board, works in a similar way to the written exercise where you document your ideal life. The main difference is, with the board, the representation is visual, which many people find more inspiring and easier to grasp and absorb, and it can be more colourful and inspiring.

Three of the main learning styles are visual, auditory and kinesthetic (touch and movement). Most people are visual which is why dream boards work so well. The idea is to embed images of the life we want to live into our subconscious mind.

The subconscious mind doesn't understand language – it thinks in feelings, emotions and images. There is no better way to combine all three than to create an inspiring visual graphic of all the things you want your life to represent and encompass.

On a deeper level, when the images on our dream board become embedded in our subconscious mind, they have a much greater chance of coming to fruition.

As an inspirational speaker and author, Abraham Hicks, says: "Every thought is powerful and any thought that is brought to mind often will eventually manifest into physical realisation".

Dream boards ensure that thoughts of what we want are always present in our minds.

If we don't have a clear vision of the life we want to live, it's like going to the supermarket without a list – you can end up with a bunch of things you didn't want or need, and forget the most important things you wanted!

The most basic way to create a dream board is to cut images from magazines or find images online and print them. Then you can stick everything on a large piece of cardboard or directly onto your wall.

Alternatively, you may create a digital version you can use as your phone or computer background. In order to ensure you are on the right track with the images you select, I recommend identifying your core values, setting your goals and writing down a vision for your life, before you start creating your dream board.

This makes it easy to select images that match your goals and vision. Here is an example of a finished product.

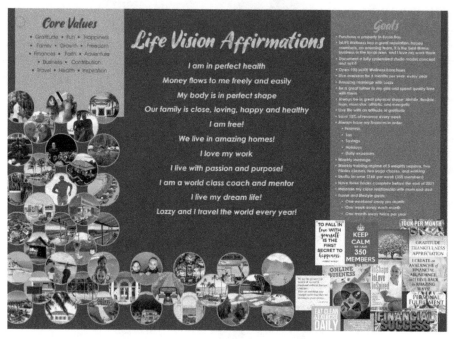

Almost every succesful person begins with two beliefs: the future can be better than the present, and I have the power to make it so.

I am fascinated with the concept of living your life doing what you love. The funny thing is, many people can't identify what they love. Where's the limitation? Money? Time? Not knowing how to do it? Not believing it's possible?

Anthony Robbins says the quality of your life depends on the quality of the questions you ask yourself. I also think if you want a better answer, then ask a better question.

How does this work in practice?

Instead of saying, "I can't do it", ask yourself, "How can I do it?"

Our mind is programmed to search for answers.

There's a part of our brain called the Reticular Activating System which is the portal through which almost all information enters our brain.

When we put the outcome we want into the universe, our Reticular Activating System goes to work, filtering and prioritising the information that is helpful for achieving our goal.

A simple example of this is when you are thinking about buying a red Mazda – then, when you're out somewhere, all you can see are red Mazdas!

Have fun with this, and then look for evidence of it working!

Set an intention to identify opportunities for a better job with fewer hours and more money, or focus on being in the best shape you can be in.

Set an intention to find the perfect partner, live your dream lifestyle, or be a loving parent.

Believe it is all possible and watch it unfold.

Dr Joe Vitale has a 5-step process for manifesting outcomes, which goes like this:

1. Think about what you don't want
2. Think about what you do want
3. Visualise it
4. Take action
5. Let it go

It's this last step that can be confusing, and it relates to being detached from the outcome. It is detachment, or allowing it to happen, or going with the flow, with the knowledge that your goal (or something better) will be achieved that dissolves the mental, emotional and spiritual barriers that we often unconsciously put up by being anxious about an outcome and stressing about things.

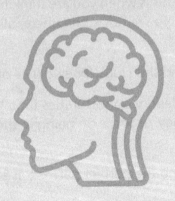

The RAS filters and prioritizes sensory information to let the mind be focused and alert.

How about some more quality questions?

How can I live my life doing what I love?

How can I make it happen?
What would this mean?
How would I feel?
How would my life be then?
What kind of person would I be?
Would I have a greater impact on the world?
Who can help me get where I want to be?
Would I be happier, more content and more fulfilled if I made some changes?
Would life be more fun and interesting?

Affirmations

Affirmations are short sentences, repeated regularly so they embed into your subconscious mind. Affirmations support and strengthen the images on our dream board. From there, with the right mental outlook and a little action, these statements eventually come to fruition.

Whether you are creating a vision for your life or writing and reading your affirmations, one key is to visualise your ideal outcomes and add positive emotion to it all.

Emotion is the language of the universe. Your subconscious mind can't tell the difference between reality and imagination, and by imagining what you desire you will align with the energetic vibration of what you want to attract and the resources, people, and events will magically be pulled into place.

is happens depends on how much you can
ocess, and release fear and doubt, which are
nce.

es:

Life Vision Affirmations

I am in perfect health
Money flows to me freely and easily
My body is in perfect shape
Our family is close, loving, happy and healthy
I am free!
We live in amazing homes!
I live with passion and purpose!
I am a world class coach and mentor
I live my dream life!
Lozzy and travel the world every year!

Design your dream life and then make it happen!

Conclusion

Thank you, and well done on completing this book. I hope it has given you some things to think about, and inspired you in some small way to want to move forward and carve out more joy and fulfilment in your life.

Please never settle for anything less than what makes you truly happy, be your best, have a go at doing something that sets your soul on fire, believe it's all possible, push through the fear, seek support, stay positive, be grateful, and have fun with it all!

"If you think you are beaten, you are
If you think you dare not, you don't,
If you like to win, but you think you can't
It is almost certain you won't.

If you think you'll lose, you're lost
For out of the world we find,
Success begins with a fellow's will
It's all in the state of mind.

If you think you are outclassed, you are
You've got to think high to rise,
You've got to be sure of yourself before
You can ever win a prize.

Life's battles don't always go
To the stronger or faster man,
But soon or late the man who wins
Is the man WHO THINKS HE CAN!"

- Walter D. Wintle

SCOTT CAPELIN

inShape inLove inSpired!